Elastography - Current Insights and Applications

Edited by Mahesh Goenka,
Akash Roy and Usha Goenka

Published in London, United Kingdom

Elastography - Current Insights and Applications
http://dx.doi.org/10.5772/intechopen.1000403
Edited by Mahesh Goenka, Akash Roy and Usha Goenka

Contributors
Akash Roy, Anant Gupta, Brian Di Giacinto, Evren Üstüner, Hector Fabio Restrepo-Guerrero, Kemal Altınbaş, Mahesh Goenka, Metin Yavuz, Sandeep Nijhawan, Usha Goenka, Yonggang Lu

Notice
Statements and opinions expressed in the chapters are these of the individual contributors and not necessarily those of the editors or publisher. No responsibility is accepted for the accuracy of information contained in the published chapters. The publisher assumes no responsibility for any damage or injury to persons or property arising out of the use of any materials, instructions, methods or ideas contained in the book.

First published in London, United Kingdom, 2025 by IntechOpen
IntechOpen is the global imprint of INTECHOPEN LIMITED, registered in England and Wales, registration number: 11086078, 167-169 Great Portland Street, London, W1W 5PF, United Kingdom

For EU product safety concerns: IN TECH d.o.o., Prolaz Marije Krucifikse Kozulić 3, 51000 Rijeka, Croatia, info@intechopen.com or visit our website at intechopen.com.

British Library Cataloguing-in-Publication Data
A catalogue record for this book is available from the British Library

Elastography - Current Insights and Applications
Edited by Mahesh Goenka, Akash Roy and Usha Goenka
p. cm.
Print ISBN 978-1-83634-230-4
Online ISBN 978-1-83634-229-8
eBook (PDF) ISBN 978-1-83634-231-1

If disposing of this product, please recycle the paper responsibly.

IntechOpen

intechopen.com

Built by scientists, for scientists

Meet the editors

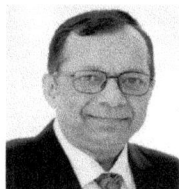

Dr. Mahesh Kumar Goenka is a senior gastroenterologist with a special interest in the field of endoscopy. He has performed over 100,000 endoscopic procedures, with expertise in advanced therapeutic endoscopy, including endoscopic retrograde cholangiopancreatography (ERCP), SpyGlass cholangioscopy, and laser lithotripsy. He is currently the Director of the Institute of Gastrosciences and Liver Transplantation, Apollo Multispeciality Hospitals, Kolkata, India. He is also a national convener for the National Board of Examinations for Medical Gastroenterology. He has over 175 publications in various books and national and international medical journals. He was the president of the Indian Society of Gastroenterology (2020–2021) and governor (Indian region) of the American College of Gastroenterology (ACG). He also served as secretary general and president of the Society of Gastrointestinal Endoscopy of India (2016–2017), for which he successfully organized the international conference, 'Asian Pacific Digestive Week 2019'. He is an honorary professor at the Medical School of Wisconsin, USA. Dr. Goenka has received multiple national and international awards, including the prestigious International Leadership Award (2020) from the American College of Gastroenterology for his contributions to gastroenterology in the international arena.

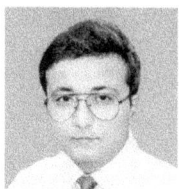

Dr. Akash Roy is a consultant hepatologist, liver transplant physician, and adjunct associate professor at Apollo Hospitals, Kolkata. He received the Professor Mindie H. Nguyen Award for Outstanding Clinical Research by an Early Career Investigator for his research on faecal microbiota transplantation in cirrhosis from the American Association for the Study of Liver Diseases (AASLD), 2002–2021. He also received the Cheung Family Memorial Travel Award for an oral presentation on original research by the AASLD Foundation in 2020. He was awarded the Best Oral Presentation at the Singapore Hepatology Conference in 2021 for his work on autoimmune hepatitis-related acute and chronic liver failure. He is the current editor of *Clinical Rounds in Hepatology*, Springer 1st Edition 2022, an Executive Editor for the *Journal of Clinical and Experimental Hepatology* and an Assistant Editor for the *Journal of Digestive Endoscopy* and *Indian Journal of Gastroenterology*. He is also a peer-reviewer for multiple international journals in hepatology. He has authored 102 research articles in national and international, peer-reviewed, indexed journals, and 27 chapters. He has also presented over 25 abstracts at national and international scientific meetings.

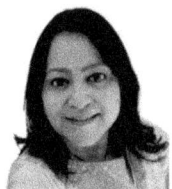

Dr. Usha Goenka is a senior interventional radiologist who specializes in vascular and nonvascular interventional radiology at the Department of Clinical Imaging and Interventional Radiology at Apollo Multispeciality Hospital, Kolkata, India. She has been a merit holder and university topper through her MBBS graduation. She completed an MD in Radiology from the prestigious Postgraduate Institute of Medical Education and Research (PGIMER), India. She has more than forty-five publications in various national and international journals. She has a keen interest in teaching and has delivered more than fifty lectures at national and international conferences. Dr. Goenka is also a member of the American College of Gastroenterology.

Contents

Preface

Elastography – Current Insights and Applications explores the guiding principles and recent developments in the field of elastography, with a focus on abdominal diseases. Elastography has seen rapid growth as a tool for evaluating multiple disease processes. The most widespread application of elastography has been in liver disease, specifically as a non-invasive tool for assessing fibrosis. However, it also finds an evolving application across many other disease entities. This book provides an overview of applications in gastrointestinal and liver disease. We explore certain bioethical principles of elastography and its application. Understanding the physical principles and techniques is crucial before embarking on elastography, as detailed in a comprehensive overview of methods. While diffuse liver disease has been well described in the literature, we look at the evolving role of elastography in focal liver lesions and assess its impact on prognostication and management. While ultrasound elastography has evolved, endoscopic ultrasound-guided elastography is also gaining acceptance, and we understand the growing applications of endoscopic ultrasound elastography, especially in pancreatic disorders. We hope this book provides readers with new vistas for understanding the core concepts of elastography and its growing avenues of application.

Mahesh Goenka and Akash Roy
Institute of Gastrosciences and Liver Transplantation,
Apollo Multispecialty Hospitals,
Kolkata, India

Usha Goenka
Department of Radiology and Imaging,
Apollo Multispecialty Hospitals,
Kolkata, India

Chapter 1

Introductory Chapter: Elastography in Gastrointestinal and Liver Disease

Akash Roy, Usha Goenka and Mahesh Goenka

1. Introduction

The gastrointestinal system encompasses various organs, including the stomach, the entire intestine, the liver, the gall bladder, the bile duct, and the pancreas. Over the past few decades, elastography has become an essential tool for assessing these organs [1]. Elastography, as a principle, is a technique to evaluate the elasticity of any tissue in response to a mechanical force [2]. It fundamentally utilizes the concept that any mechanical force will cause a change or perturbation of a tissue, and that change can be analyzed to understand the inherent biomechanical properties of the tissue [2, 3]. Many different modalities exist to measure elastography, including strain elastography, shear wave elastography, and magnetic resonance elastography [2, 3]. Overall, most of the modalities aim to calculate the speed of a particular shear wave. The calculated speed is then converted to conventional Young's modulus to ascertain tissue stiffness. One of the principal advantages of elastography lies in its non-invasive nature and ease of performance [4].

2. The expanding field of elastography in liver diseases

The widest application of elastography in gastrointestinal diseases has been in hepatology. Assessing liver fibrosis using invasive liver biopsy has long been the gold standard [5]. However, liver biopsy has inherent risks of complications like bleeding, and hence, non-invasive techniques have become popular as means for fibrosis assessment [5]. Transient elastography has become a globally available and standardized tool for non-invasive fibrosis assessment [6]. Besides fibrosis assessment, the use of elastography has expanded further in other fields of hepatology. The degree of liver stiffness measurement has been used to predict clinically significant portal hypertension, presence of varices, prediction for decompensating events, and as measures of response to therapy [6]. Furthermore, dynamic changes in elastography are becoming increasingly popular as a prognostic tool to predict progression and regression of disease [7]. Very recently, severity stratification using liver stiffness measurements of liver disease has been suggested using the "rule of five" [8]. Additionally, metrics of change of liver stiffness measurement, which reflect actual changes of significance, have also been proposed [8].

IntechOpen

While transient elastography has been widely established and is more accessible, other modalities of liver elastography have also been explored. Ultrasound-based measures using point shear wave elastography, acoustic radiation forced impulse, and 2D shear wave elastography provide readily reportable tools for radiologists performing conventional ultrasounds [9]. Recent efforts have been made to validate and standardize various ultrasound-based techniques, and specific guidelines have been laid down for the same [10]. A more advanced and extremely accurate technique utilizes the use of magnetic resonance elastography to ascertain tissue stiffness [11]. It has been found to reflect closely on biopsy measures of fibrosis and is especially beneficial in obese patients, where transient elastography and ultrasound elastography may have technical difficulties and challenges. Like transient elastography, magnetic resonance elastography has also been used to predict varices and decompensation in individuals with cirrhosis [11, 12]. While all elastography techniques have become popular and widely available, it is also important to understand the limitations of elastography [13]. Transient elastography is limited in the presence of severe obesity. It is not reliable in the presence of ascites or acute hepatitis with aminotransferase levels of more than five times the upper limit of normal [14]. Also, interpretation needs to be done with caution in patients with the features of congestive heart failure and chronic kidney disease on dialysis. MR elastography, on the other hand, is limited in the presence of severe iron deposition and ascites and is challenging in those with claustrophobia [14]. Hence, for any elastographic technique, the clinicians' decision-making and interpretation are of key importance.

Besides fibrosis assessment, a few other emerging fields are ascertaining elastographic features in space-occupying lesions to differentiate benign and malignant lesions and identifying unique elastographic signatures of malignant space-occupying lesions [15]. Estimating muscle stiffness with elastography in patients with cirrhosis is also an emerging field [16]. Hence, elastographic techniques in liver disease have already established themselves as essential tools and are an expanding field.

3. Evolution of pancreatic elastography

Pancreatic elastography allows the assessment of pancreatic tissue stiffness by virtual palpation. It is mainly done using two main types of techniques: pancreatic strain elastography, applied by endoscopic ultrasound, which has been used to characterize small solid pancreatic lesions, and shear wave elastography, which has a more limited but evolving role in larger solid pancreatic lesions [17]. The use of elastography in pancreatic diseases has also been found to be applicable in the characterization of chronic pancreatitis, autoimmune pancreatitis, and disorders like pancreatic tuberculosis [18]. It has also been seen that in cases of acute pancreatitis, necrotic tissues appear less stiff than the surrounding parenchyma [18]. The characterization of solid pancreatic lesions is based upon whether the lesion is more or less stiff compared to the surrounding parenchyma. These principles have been used in characterizing pancreatic ductal adenocarcinoma, pancreatic neuroendocrine tumors, and mass-forming pancreatitis [17, 18]. Recent efforts have also been made to improve the reproducibility, accuracy, and clinical utility of elastography in pancreatic imaging, which have moved toward developing quantitative scoring systems for elastography to delineate better the relative differences in the elasticity of solid pancreatic masses [19]. The field of pancreatic elastography continues to emerge as an extremely useful tool in the hands of gastroenterologists dealing with complex pancreatic solid lesions as well as parenchymal pathologies.

4. Evolving applications in intestinal pathologies

Another evolving field is the use of ultrasound in ascertaining intestinal pathologies. In this context, ultrasound-based elastography has been shown to be an innovative, non-invasive, readily available, ancillary technique in the evaluation of intestinal fibrosis as a monitorable biomarker, in terms of stiffness [20]. Preliminary data from patients with Crohn's disease and ulcerative colitis indicate intestinal ultrasound and tissue stiffness as a potential surrogate indicator of histological fibrosis [20]. However, the field is in its incipient stages, and literature continues to evolve.

Overall, elastographic techniques have evolved to be an excellent tool in the hands of radiologists, hepatologists, and gastroenterologists in multiple gastrointestinal diseases and remain an exciting area for future research.

Conflicts of interest

None.

Author details

Akash Roy[1], Usha Goenka[2] and Mahesh Goenka[1*]

1 Institute of Gastrosciences and Liver Transplant, Apollo Multispeciality Hospitals, Kolkata, India

2 Department of Radiology and Imaging, Apollo Multispeciality Hospitals, Kolkata, India

*Address all correspondence to: mkgkolkata@gmail.com

IntechOpen

References

[1] Havre R, Gilja OH. Elastography and strain rate imaging of the gastrointestinal tract. European Journal of Radiology. 2014;**83**(3):438-441

[2] Garra BS. Elastography: History, principles, and technique comparison. Abdominal Imaging. 2015;**40**:680-697

[3] Barr RG. Elastography in clinical practice. Radiologic Clinics. 2014;**52**(6):1145-1162

[4] Hoskins PR. Principles of ultrasound elastography. Ultrasound. 2012;**20**(1):8-15

[5] Bravo AA, Sheth SG, Chopra S. Liver biopsy. New England Journal of Medicine. 2001;**344**(7):495-500

[6] Jung KS, Kim SU. Clinical applications of transient elastography. Clinical and Molecular Hepatology. 2012;**18**(2):163

[7] Leite NC, Villela-Nogueira CA, Santos LV, Cardoso CR, Salles GF. Prognostic value of changes in vibration-controlled transient elastography parameters for liver, cardiovascular and mortality outcomes in individuals with type 2 diabetes and metabolic dysfunction-associated steatotic liver disease: The Rio de Janeiro type 2 diabetes cohort. Diabetes, Obesity and Metabolism. 2025;**27**(4):2024-2034

[8] Mendizabal M, Cançado GG, Albillos A. Evolving portal hypertension through Baveno VII recommendations. Annals of Hepatology. 2024;**29**(1):101180

[9] Ye J, Huang Y, Sun Y, Shao C, Zhang S, Wang W, et al. Dynamic monitoring with shear wave elastography predicts outcomes of chronic hepatitis B patients with decompensated cirrhosis. Annals of Translational Medicine. 2021;**9**(21):1613

[10] Ferraioli G, Barr RG, Berzigotti A, Sporea I, Wong VW, Reiberger T, et al. WFUMB guideline/guidance on liver multiparametric ultrasound: Part 1. Update to 2018 guidelines on liver ultrasound elastography. Ultrasound in Medicine & Biology. 2024;**50**(8):1071-1087. DOI: 10.1016/j.ultrasmedbio.2024.03.013

[11] Selvaraj EA, Mózes FE, Jayaswal AN, Zafarmand MH, Vali Y, Lee JA, et al. Diagnostic accuracy of elastography and magnetic resonance imaging in patients with NAFLD: A systematic review and meta-analysis. Journal of Hepatology. 2021;**75**(4):770-785

[12] Roy A, Verma N, Jajodia S, Goenka U, Tiwari A, Sonthalia N, et al. Magnetic resonance elastography (MRE) outperforms acoustic force radiation impulse (ARFI) in predicting oesophageal varices in obese NAFLD cirrhosis. Abdominal Radiology. 2024;**49**(9):3088-3095

[13] Oglat AA, Abukhalil T. Ultrasound Elastography: Methods, clinical applications, and limitations: A review article. Applied Sciences. 2024;**14**(10):4308

[14] Villani R, Lupo P, Sangineto M, Romano AD, Serviddio G. Liver ultrasound elastography in non-alcoholic fatty liver disease: A state-of-the-art summary. Diagnostics. 2023;**13**(7):1236

[15] Guo J, Jiang D, Qian Y, Yu J, Gu YJ, Zhou YQ, et al. Differential diagnosis of different types of solid focal liver lesions using two-dimensional shear

wave elastography. World Journal of Gastroenterology. 2022;**28**(32):4716

[16] Becchetti C, Lange NF, Delgado MG, Brönnimann MP, Maurer MH, Dufour JF, et al. 2D shear wave elastography of the rectus femoris muscle in patients with cirrhosis: Feasibility and clinical findings. A pilot study. Clinics and Research in Hepatology and Gastroenterology. 2023;**47**(3):102080

[17] Dietrich CF, Hocke M. Elastography of the pancreas, current view. Clinical Endoscopy. 2019;**52**(6):533-540

[18] Goertz RS, Schuderer J, Strobel D, Pfeifer L, Neurath MF, Wildner D. Acoustic radiation force impulse shear wave elastography (ARFI) of acute and chronic pancreatitis and pancreatic tumor. European Journal of Radiology. 2016;**85**:2211

[19] Săftoiu A, Vilmann P, Gorunescu F, et al. Accuracy of endoscopic ultrasound elastography used for differential diagnosis of focal pancreatic masses: A multicenter study. Endoscopy. 2011;**43**:596-603

[20] Dal Buono A, Faita F, Peyrin-Biroulet L, Danese S, Allocca M. Ultrasound elastography in inflammatory bowel diseases: A systematic review of accuracy compared with histopathological assessment. Journal of Crohn's and Colitis. 2022;**16**(10):1637-1646

Chapter 2

Physical Principles and Imaging Techniques of Ultrasound Elastography

Yonggang Lu and Brian Di Giacinto

Abstract

In this chapter, the physical principles of ultrasound elastography are introduced, followed by a description of two fundamental ultrasound-based elastography imaging techniques: strain elastography and shear wave elastography. For these two techniques, their basic mechanisms, implementation strategies, advantages, and limitations are compared. Image quality and artifacts along with improvement methods in elastographies are also examined, followed by emphasizing the bioeffects and safety of each elastography technique. Finally, issues related to quality assurance in elastography, such as machine calibration, system performance testing, the use of phantoms, standardization of acquisition protocols, inter-operator, and intra-operator variability, as well as regulatory standards and guidelines, are discussed.

Keywords: ultrasound elastography, physical principles, imaging techniques, image quality and artifact, bioeffect and safety, quality assurance

1. Introduction

Ultrasound Elastography (USE) is a cutting-edge imaging technology that has revolutionized the ability to non-invasively assess mechanical properties of human tissues, particularly their stiffness [1, 2]. This method offers clinicians unique real-time insight into patient health and active surveillance of chronic disease by capitalizing on the changes in tissue stiffness that accompany pathologic processes, such as fibrosis, inflammation, and cellular depletion or proliferation induced by musculoskeletal disorders, neoplasia, and chronic liver disease [3–6]. The principle behind USE is straightforward: soft tissues, like normal liver tissue, deform more readily when subjected to mechanical forces, whereas stiffer tissues, such as those affected by tumors or fibrosis, are more resistant to deformation. Modern elastography techniques provide methods and tools to evaluate and quantify tissue stiffness [7, 8].

This chapter will delve into the physical principles of ultrasound elastography and explore various elastography techniques including their advantages and limitations, relevant artifacts, bioeffects, safety considerations, and elastography specific quality assurance measures to lay a foundation for understanding and utilizing this powerful diagnostic modality.

IntechOpen

2. Physical principles of ultrasound elastography

2.1 Tissue mechanics

Understanding the mechanical properties of tissues and how they influence an organs response to both internal and external forces is fundamental to ultrasound elastography. The key parameters that describe how tissues deform include stress, strain, elasticity, and viscoelasticity. Ultrasound elastography leverages these parameters to measure and present visual maps of tissue stiffness [7, 9].

2.1.1 Stress and strain

Stress (σ) is defined as the force (F) applied per unit area (A) of tissue ($\sigma = F / A$), typically expressed in Pascals ($Pa = N / m^2$). Strain (ε) refers to the deformation or displacement that occurs as a result of applied stress [7]. It is a dimensionless quantity that measures the relative change in shape or size of interrogated tissue (l), i.e.,

$$\varepsilon = \Delta l / l \tag{1}$$

In elastography, tissue strain is measured or estimated after applying a force, either external compression or through the generation of internal shear waves [1, 9]. Relatively soft tissues, such as normal muscle, fat, or liver, generally exhibit greater strain under a given stress compared to stiffer tissues, such as a cirrhotic liver or a fibrous hypercellular neoplasm [3].

2.1.2 Elasticity and modulus

Elasticity is the ability of a material or substance to return to its original shape after deformation with the assumption of non-compressibility. USE relies heavily on the concept of tissue elasticity. Different tissues exhibit different elastic properties. The elastic behavior of tissues can be described quantitatively using elastic modulus (Γ), which is a measure of stiffness. It represents the ratio of stress to strain (Pa), i.e.,

$$\Gamma = \sigma / \varepsilon \tag{2}$$

The velocity (c) of elastic waves in tissue is related to its density (ρ) and elastic modulus (Eq. (3)). Most forms of elastography leverage this relationship to calculate tissue stiffness under the assumption that the tissue being measured is homogenously dense, isotropic, and purely elastic. Specifically, the velocity of an ultrasound wave through tissue is measured and the modulus is subsequently calculated by assuming tissue density is equal to water:

$$\Gamma = \rho c^2 \rightarrow c = \sqrt{\frac{\Gamma}{\rho}} \tag{3}$$

There are various elastic moduli. Young's modulus (E) is one of the moduli which denotes the tissue change under compressive or tensile stress, defined to be the ratio of compressive/tensile stress (σ_n) to compressive/tensile strain (ε_n):

$$E = \sigma_n / \varepsilon_n \qquad (4)$$

Shear modulus (G) is another modulus which describes how tissues change under shear stress. It is defined as the ratio of shear stress (σ_s) to shear strain (ε_s).

$$G = \sigma_s / \varepsilon_s \qquad (5)$$

While Young's modulus describes how a material responds to compressive or tensile stress, the shear modulus describes how a tissue resists shear forces, where layers of the tissue are displaced relative to each other (**Figure 1**).

Young's modulus in tissue is related to shear modulus through Poisson's ratio (ν):

$$E = 2G(1 + \nu) \qquad (6)$$

Poisson's ratio equals 0.5 for soft biological tissues that are assumed to be noncompressible and isotropic (**Figure 2**) [2]. Therefore, the relationship between Young's modulus and shear modulus is given by:

$$E = 2G(1 + \nu) = 3G \qquad (7)$$

Thus, Young's modulus is equal to about three times shear modulus for most human tissues [1].

2.1.3 Nonlinear elasticity

Biological tissues often exhibit nonlinear elasticity, meaning their mechanical response to stress is not proportional to the applied force. In other words, as tissues are subjected to increasing levels of stress, their stiffness may change (**Figure 3**). This is particularly important in elastography because tissues may behave differently under low versus high levels of compression or shear forces.

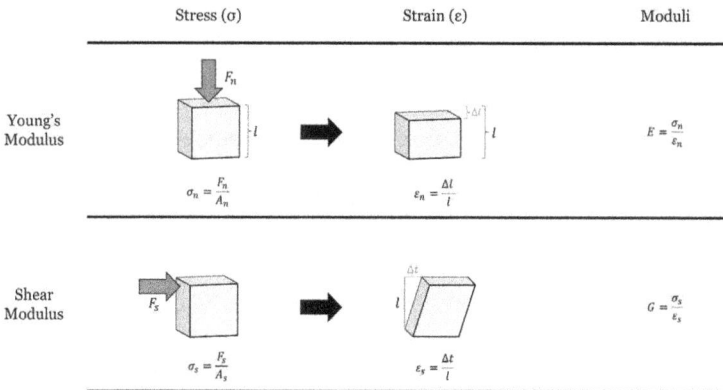

Figure 1.
Young's modulus (E) and shear modulus (G).

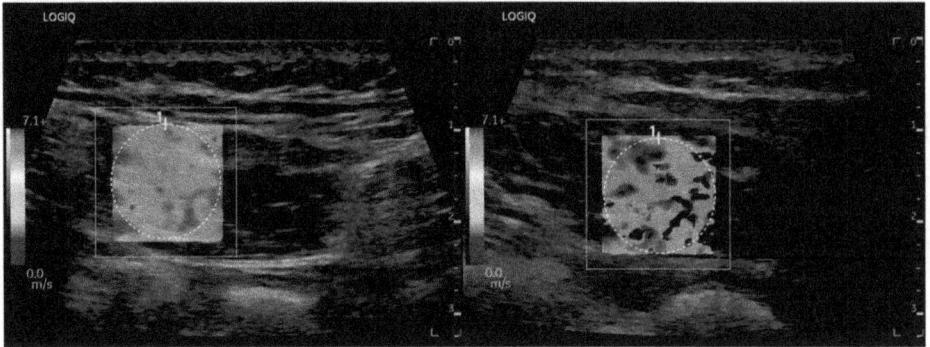

Figure 2.
2D shear wave elastography of the inferior abdominus rectus muscle with gray scale and color elastogram on a GE LOGIQ 10 system with a L2-9 transducer. Shear waves traveling perpendicular to the muscle fibers (left) are slower than shear waves traveling parallel to the muscle fibers (right).

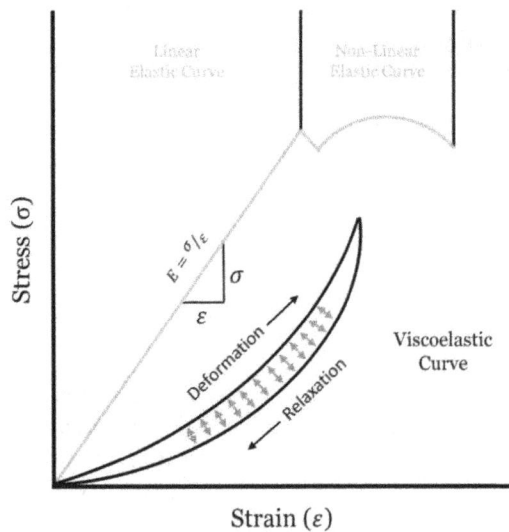

Figure 3.
Stress-strain curve comparing the linear and non-linear portions of a strictly elastic substance (blue) with a viscoelastic substance (black). Note the difference in between deformation and relaxation curves of a viscoelastic substance due to dissipation of heat (red double arrows).

For example, normal tissues may exhibit low stiffness at low stress levels but become stiffer as the applied stress increases. Conversely, pathological tissues like tumors may start out stiff and show little change in stiffness even under high stress. Nonlinear elasticity is a key consideration in techniques such as strain elastography, where tissue response to compression can vary depending on the amount of force applied [10].

2.1.4 Viscoelasticity

Biological tissues exhibit viscoelastic properties, meaning they combine both elastic (solid-like) and viscous (fluid-like) behaviors. In purely elastic materials, deformation is instantaneous and fully reversible when stress is applied or removed. However, in viscoelastic tissues, the response to stress is time-dependent, meaning deformation occurs over time and some energy is dissipated as heat during deformation (**Figure 3**). In practice, tissues like liver, kidney, muscle, and breast are viscoelastic.

Viscoelastic properties are crucial in elastography. Especially in dynamic elastography techniques like shear wave elastography, where the tissue's response to time-varying stresses is evaluated. In pathological tissues like tumors or fibrotic areas, the viscoelastic properties are altered with time varying stress which corresponds to higher stiffness. Ultrasound elastography typically assumes elastic properties, which may lead to inaccuracies in viscoelastic tissues [9, 10].

2.1.5 Anisotropy

Anisotropy refers to the directional dependence of mechanical properties, such as resistance to flow or response to compressive, tensile, or shearing forces. USE assumes that the sampled tissue responds to stress isotropically, meaning that tissue strain would be identical regardless of the orientation of the applied stress. In practice, however, some tissues will deform differently depending on the orientation of applied stress. Muscles and ligaments are highly anisotropic as they are comprised of long bundled cylindrical fascicles running the entire length from origin to insertion [11]. They are highly resistant to tensile and compressive stresses applied parallel to the fibers but deform readily to stresses applied perpendicular to the fibers. Kidneys are also highly anisotropic due to the radial orientation of the tubules, collecting ducts, and vasa recta from the renal sinus. When the ultrasound beam is oriented perpendicular to the capsule and along the tubules the shear waves generated from the beam will travel perpendicularly through the radially oriented tubules. The numerous interfaces slow the shear waves, artificially reducing the measured stiffness of the renal parenchyma [12, 13].

In elastography, anisotropy can complicate stiffness measurements because tissue strain and shear wave propagation speed may vary depending on the orientation of the tissue. Advanced elastography techniques are being developed to account for anisotropy by measuring tissue stiffness in multiple directions (2D or 3D), providing a more comprehensive picture of tissue mechanics [11, 14].

2.2 Shear wave

2.2.1 Shear wave generation and propagation

Shear waves are transverse waves where particle motion is perpendicular to the direction of wave propagation. Conversely, in longitudinal waves, particle motion is parallel to the direction of wave propagation, as shown in **Figure 4**. There are two common approaches to generate shear waves in tissues:

a. Acoustic radiation force impulse (ARFI): A short, high-intensity focused ultrasound pulse which can induce localized displacements of tissue with longitudinal waves to generate shear waves propagating from the focal point.

b. External mechanical vibration: This involves mechanically vibrating the target tissue with low frequency sound waves, a vibrating plate, or a passive driver to introduce shear waves in tissue.

Shear waves decay relatively quickly as they propagate through tissue because they are rapidly attenuated, especially in soft tissues. The rate of attenuation is dependent

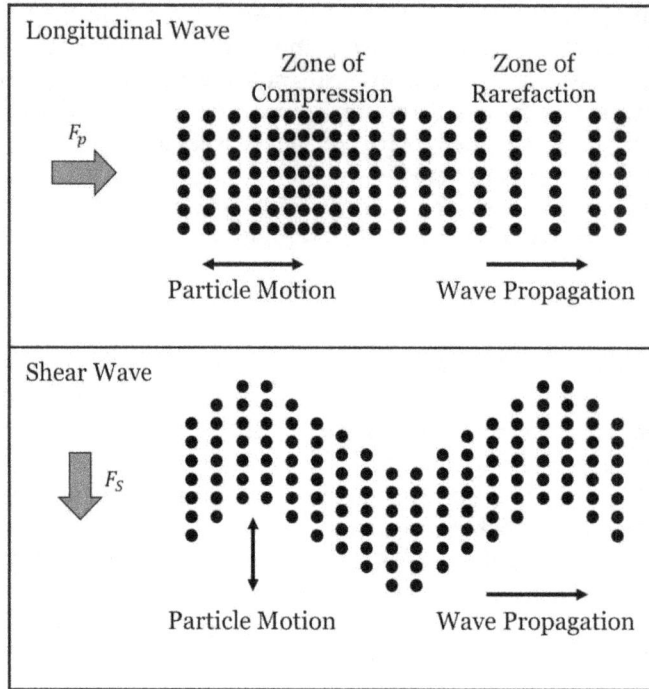

Figure 4.
Propagation of longitudinal and shear waves.

on tissue's viscoelastic properties. In complex, heterogeneous tissues (like liver, kidney, or muscle), shear waves may exhibit scattering or refraction, which makes advanced processing techniques necessary to reconstruct accurate stiffness maps [1, 10].

2.2.2 Shear wave detection and measurement

After the shear waves are generated, the ultrasound system uses cross-correlation or phase-sensitive techniques to track tissue displacements caused by the shear waves. High-frame-rate longitudinal ultrasound imaging (thousands of frames per second) is employed to visualize the propagation of the shear wavefronts through tissue in real-time. Shear wave speed is calculated by measuring the time it takes for the shear wave to travel over a known distance.

Shear waves typically propagate through soft tissue at speeds between 1 and 10 m/s, much slower than the longitudinal waves (approximately 1540 m/s in soft tissues) used to track them. The stiffer the tissue, the faster shear waves move [9].

3. Ultrasound elastography imaging techniques

Ultrasound elastography can be classified by differences in measured physical quantity, excitation method, and method of displaying the measured quantity. In this chapter, we classify elastography techniques into two fundamental categories: strain elastography and shear wave elastography. Regardless of the manufacturer's name or proprietary excitation method, all ultrasound elastography is ultimately derivative of these two techniques. Implementation strategies, advantages, and limitations of both techniques will be discussed.

3.1 Strain elastography

3.1.1 Basic mechanism

Strain elastography (SE) applies a compressive force (either manual compression, physiological movements, or acoustic radiation force impulse) to deform the tissue. The tissue displacement is tracked and calculated by comparing pre-compression and post-compression ultrasound images. The tissue's deformation (strain) is then computed based on these displacements. An elastogram is presented as a color map of relative strain magnitude layered over a B-mode image (**Figure 5**).

3.1.2 Implementation strategies

3.1.2.1 Technical workflow

1. Pre-compression image acquisition: A baseline ultrasound image is obtained before applying any mechanical force.

2. Compression: Mechanical force is applied through either manual compression, physiological movements, or acoustic radiation force impulse.

3. Post-compression image acquisition: A second ultrasound image is taken after applying force.

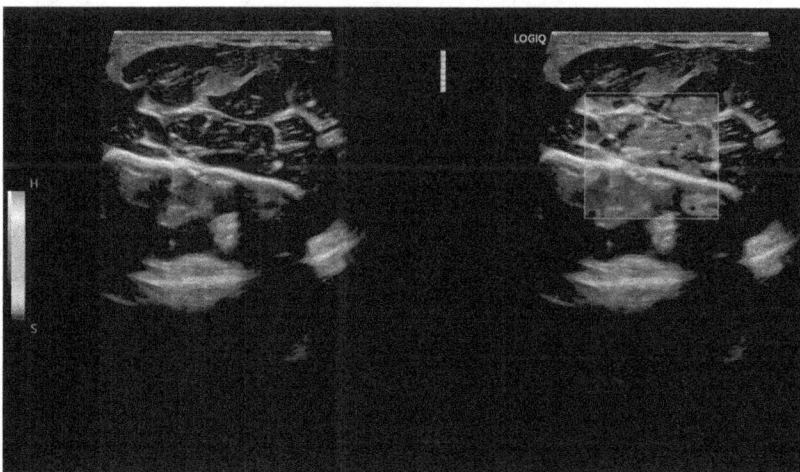

Figure 5.
Strain elastography of the forearm with gray scale and color elastogram using manual compression on a GE LOGIQ 10 system with a L2-9 transducer. B-mode image (left) shows the anterior compartments of the left forearm, radius, ulna, and interosseous membrane. Elastogram (right) with a color scale (red: hard, blue: soft) exhibits the markedly increased stiffness of the bones and interosseous membrane relative to the musculature of the anterior compartment.

4. Displacement measurement: Tissue displacement between the two images is calculated using cross-correlation or phase-sensitive techniques.

5. Strain calculation: The relative deformation (strain) is computed and an elastogram is generated.

6. Image interpretation: Clinicians interpret the elastogram to evaluate tissue stiffness.

3.1.2.2 Key techniques

Force application methods: There are three main ways to apply mechanical force to the tissue in strain elastography:

- Manual compression: The ultrasound operator applies cyclic compression and decompression on the body surface with the ultrasound transducer. The degree of deformation depends on how much pressure is applied, and this method is operator dependent.

- Physiological motion: Natural body movements such as heartbeat or breathing are used to induce strain. This is more common in certain applications, such as in cardiac elastography.

- Acoustic radiation force impulse (ARFI): ARFI imaging does not rely on transducer compression and has the advantage of being able to focus the 'push' within deep lying organs, where it can be difficult to generate deformation with compression from the body surface.

With respect to manual compression of the body surface, it is possible to apply pressure up to the normal diagnostic depth of superficial organs such as the breast and thyroid gland; however, stress is not easily transmitted to deep organs such as the liver, making it difficult to elicit strain. Therefore, strain induced by either cardiovascular pulsation or respiration is used for evaluation of liver fibrosis with strain imaging.

Strain calculation: The ultrasound system searches for corresponding points between frames of pre-compression and post-compression ultrasound images, using ultrasound signals. The displacement of the tissue is tracked by analyzing the changes in the ultrasound signals using a cross-correlation method or phase-sensitive techniques. Once displacement is calculated, strain is derived by calculating the spatial derivative of the displacement field.

Elastogram creation: A color-coded map of tissue stiffness known as a color elastogram is generated based on the magnitude of strain. It is common to superimpose a translucent colored elastogram atop the B-mode image. At present, no standardized color map exists. In most equipment, users can select the color scale as desired. The color mapping is qualitative and gives a visual sense of tissue stiffness.

Noise reduction and image smoothing: Because small tissue displacements are often used, noise reduction techniques such as temporal filtering, spatial smoothing, and adaptive algorithms are applied to improve image quality and reduce artifacts.

Analysis: Strain elastography typically does not provide quantitative values for stiffness but rather a relative comparison between tissues within the region of interest

(ROI). Some systems can provide semi-quantitative measurements by comparing the stiffness of an ROI to a reference tissue or by calculating the strain ratio between two regions (e.g., lesion vs. surrounding normal tissue). Higher ratios suggest that the lesion is stiffer relative to the surrounding tissue.

Variants of strain elastography: There are several approaches to strain elastography, each with unique technical details:

- Static strain elastography: It involves applying manual compression to the tissue and capturing images before and after the compression to assess strain. It is useful for characterizing lesions in breast and thyroid tissues [15].

- Dynamic strain elastography: It applies continuous or periodic mechanical forces to the tissue, allowing for real-time strain measurement. It is often used for evaluating deeper structures like the liver [16].

- Real-time elastography: It provides immediate assessment of tissue stiffness during the ultrasound exam, using a visual color-coded map to indicate strain. This technique is commonly used in liver studies to assess fibrosis [17].

- Acoustic radiation force impulse imaging: Focused ultrasound beams create localized shear waves, and the displacement is measured to assess tissue stiffness. This technique is commonly used to evaluate stiffness of liver and kidney [18].

3.1.3 Limitations and considerations

- *Operator dependency*: One of the major limitations of strain elastography is its reliance on operator skill, especially when manual compression is used. Inconsistent compression often causes increased stiffness of the background tissue and increases elastogram variability.

- *Qualitative nature*: Strain elastography normally does not provide quantitative stiffness measurements, only a qualitative comparison of stiffness relative to adjacent tissues.

- *Tissue homogeneity assumptions*: Strain elastography assumes tissue homogeneity, which is often not the case in real biological tissues.

3.2 Shear wave elastography

3.2.1 Basic mechanism

In shear wave elastography (SWE), shear waves are generated within the tissue using an ARFI or external mechanical vibrator. The longitudinal ultrasound beam pushes on the tissue, causing localized displacement in targeted regions of interest (ROIs). The tissue's response to this displacement leads to the generation of shear waves which propagate perpendicularly to the ultrasound beam. Shear wave speed is then measured using cross-correlation or phase-sensitive techniques. Shear modulus or Young's modulus is then calculated based on the measured shear wave speed. Either shear wave speed or one of the calculated elastic moduli are then presented as a color map overlaid on B-mode image and quantified as numerical metrics (**Figure 6**).

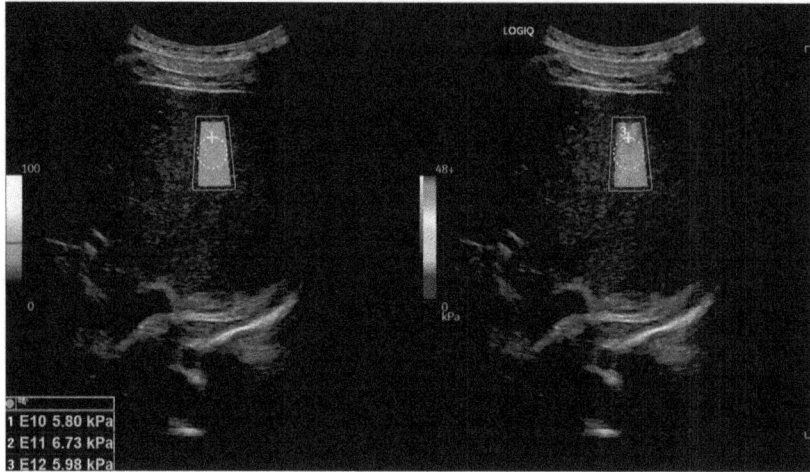

Figure 6.
A SWE elastogram of the liver on a GE LOGIQ 10 system which is based on the ARFI imaging technique (with a C1-6 transducer). B-mode US image with overlaid quality map (left) and overlaid color map of simultaneous shear wave measurements (right).

3.2.2 Implementation strategies

3.2.2.1 Technical workflow

1. Preliminary ultrasound imaging: Standard ultrasound imaging is first performed to localize the area of interest.

2. Shear wave generation: Acoustic radiation force or external mechanical force is applied.

3. Shear wave detection: High-frame-rate ultrasound imaging tracks the shear wave propagation.

4. Stiffness calculation: The shear wave speed is measured, and often shear or Young's modulus is calculated.

5. Elastogram display: A color-coded stiffness map (elastogram) is displayed, showing tissue stiffness or shear wave speed in real-time.

3.2.2.2 Key techniques

Shear wave generation (for ARFI): Acoustic radiation force impulse is applied at a single focal location or a multiple focal zone configuration in which each focal zone is interrogated in rapid succession, leading to a cylindrically shaped shear wave extending over a larger depth, enabling real-time shear wave images to be formed.

Shear wave detection and tracking: SWE uses high-frame-rate ultrasound imaging to capture the shear wave motion in real-time, often at frame rates of several thousand frames per second. The key steps include:

1. Ultrasound pulse echoes: The system sends conventional ultrasound pulses to create an image of tissue and detect the tissue's displacement.

2. Cross-correlation: Tissue displacement is calculated using a cross-correlation method between the pre- and post-push ultrasound frames. This allows the system to measure the time it takes for the shear wave to travel a known distance, giving the shear wave velocity.

Advanced signal processing: SWE involves sophisticated signal processing, to handle fast acquisition and processing of data, such as using temporal filtering, spatial smoothing, noise reduction, and artifact reduction. Inversion algorithms are especially helpful to reconstruct the tissue's stiffness properties based on the measured wave propagation data, accounting for factors like attenuation and tissue heterogeneity to improve reconstruction accuracy.

Elastogram creation: SWE generates a quantitative color-coded elastogram map, where each pixel corresponds to a stiffness value in shear wave velocity (m/s), shear modulus, or Young's modulus (kPa).

Variants of SWE: There are several approaches to shear wave elastography, each with unique technical details:

- Point SWE: This version of SWE measures the shear wave speed at a single point, often used for assessing specific organs like liver. It gives a continuous numerical stiffness value at a small ROI. The ROI size is a tradeoff between precision and spatial resolution in shear wave speed estimation methods. The use of larger propagation distances to compute the wave speed presumes a larger homogeneous region and typically is associated with higher precision and accuracy; however, this comes at the expense of spatial resolution. This technique can provide real time and quantitative stiffness measurements of very small structures by evaluating tissue stiffness only at a single focal point. However, depth of penetration is limited with point SWE and more measurements are usually required due to increased noise and measurement variability [19]. This can be challenging for patients with cardiorespiratory disease or large volume ascites as a prolonged breath-hold is often required to complete elastogram acquisition.

- 2D SWE: This is the most common SWE technique in research and radiology applications. It provides a 2D elastogram over a broader area, allowing for more rapid and comprehensive tissue assessment. To generate two-dimensional shear wave images, smaller propagation distances are utilized to obtain better spatial resolution; however, decreasing the distance over which the shear wave is monitored increases the variance of the estimate at each pixel. Resolution of 1–2 mm has been reported for shear wave imaging systems. 2D SWE offers a significant advantage over point-based methods by providing a broader, faster, more comprehensive assessment of tissue stiffness. Less samples are required to achieve consistent measurements. However, 2D-SWE is still limited by depth of penetration as the longitudinal waves used to generate and track shear waves are rapidly attenuated at depth [20].

- 3D SWE: This technique allows for volumetric assessment of tissue stiffness. 3D SWE offers a more comprehensive and detailed assessment of tissue stiffness, making it a valuable tool for detecting and characterizing complex or heterogeneous conditions. 3D elastography is also less impacted by artifact from anisotropic tissues. It is particularly useful in breast imaging, musculoskeletal assessment, and cancer detection. However, its cost, complexity, and longer acquisition and processing times are notable drawbacks that limit widespread adoption in most healthcare settings [14, 21].

- 4D SWE: The development of four-dimensional (real-time 3D) shear wave elastography provides dynamic volumetric information about tissue stiffness over time. 4D SWE has the potential to revolutionize how certain diseases are diagnosed and monitored, particularly those involving dynamic tissues, such as the heart, lungs, and muscles. However, given high cost and limited commercial availability, 4D SWE is not yet widely implemented in routine clinical practice. Its use is mainly confined to research settings or specialized centers. As research progresses and technology matures, 4D SWE could become an essential tool in specialized clinical applications [22].

- Multifrequency SWE: This method offers the ability to assess tissue mechanical properties more comprehensively by analyzing how different tissue types respond to a spectrum of frequencies. Different frequencies allow for better depth penetration and contrast or spatial resolution. Higher frequencies produce superior superficial tissues but are attenuated rapidly. Lower frequencies penetrate deeper into tissues. Utilizing a broad spectrum of frequencies simultaneously allows more complete assessment of tissue properties with higher spatial resolution at multiple depths, improving diagnostic accuracy. However, its increased complexity, cost, and the need for more clinical validation limits its widespread adoption in the short term [23].

- Ultrasound transient elastography (UTE): Ultrasound based transient elastography applies a series of external mechanical vibrations with low-frequency (typically in the range of 50 Hz) mechanical pulses for short durations (transient) at the skin surface then measures the tissue displacement using M-mode US. UTE is relatively operator independent. The automated nature of the test reduces variability caused by operator error, ensuring consistent readings between clinicians. However, unlike 2D shear wave elastography, UTE provides a single, global stiffness value averaged over a very large ROI and no grayscale imaging is produced to guarantee measurement of the desired tissue. This reduces accuracy and limits application of UTE to large organs with predictable positions near the skin surface. Thus, UTE is primarily designed for liver stiffness assessment and has limited application in other organs. It does not provide comprehensive information for other tissues or conditions, greatly limiting its versatility [24].

- Supersonic shear imaging (SSI): A variation of SWE, SSI involves the generation of a Mach cone (a supersonic wavefront) by rapidly moving the ultrasound focus. This allows for faster shear wave generation and greater tissue coverage in real-time. SSI uses shear waves that can penetrate deeper into tissues, making it suitable for imaging deeper organs and providing reliable stiffness measurements even in deeper tissue layers. However, SSI systems are expensive compared to other elastography techniques and less readily available compared to other USE methods. The advanced hardware requirements, combined with the integration of real-time imaging and high-speed data acquisition, increases the overall cost, limiting its availability to certain clinical settings [25].

- Time harmonic elastography (THE): THE integrates multifrequency tissue harmonic imaging with elastography to reduce artifact and improve contrast resolution at depth. Limited research suggests that THE can assess deep tissues with greater contrast resolution than other elastography methods while simultaneously generating grayscale imaging and whole organ elastograms. If confirmed in larger trials this would make THE useful for evaluating small deep organs like the adrenal glands, inconsistently positioned organs like the kidneys, and even more superficial organ in patients with very high BMI, a patient population that is currently very challenging to evaluate with USE. THE is currently limited to specialized centers and research facilities due to the cost and specialized equipment required at this stage of development [26].

3.2.3 Advantages and limitations

Advantages of Shear Wave Elastography:

- Quantitative measurement: Unlike strain elastography, which mostly provides qualitative data, SWE provides quantitative values for tissue stiffness in or kPa.

- Non-operator dependent: Since SWE relies on automatic generation of shear waves through acoustic radiation force, it is less dependent on the skill and experience of the operator compared to manual techniques like strain elastography.

- Real-time imaging: SWE can provide real-time feedback, which is helpful for live monitoring of tissue stiffness during medical procedures or follow-up examinations.

- Wide dynamic range: SWE has a wide range of stiffness measurements, making it useful for various tissue types and pathologies.

Limitations of Shear Wave Elastography:

- Attenuation in deep tissues: Shear waves attenuate quickly, especially in soft and deeper tissues. This limits the depth at which SWE can be applied effectively, particularly in obese patients or in deep-seated organs.

- Tissue heterogeneity: Tissues that are non-homogeneous, such as those containing fibrosis, fat, or calcifications, may cause wave scattering or refraction, making the stiffness measurements less reliable in certain cases.

- Viscoelastic behavior: Biological tissues are often viscoelastic, meaning their mechanical properties depend on the frequency of the applied force. SWE typically assumes elastic properties, which may lead to inaccuracies in viscoelastic tissues.

4. Image quality and artifacts of elastography

Image quality and the presence of artifacts in ultrasound elastography are critical factors that influence the diagnostic accuracy and reliability of tissue stiffness measurements. Several factors can affect the quality of elastographic images, including the imaging technique used, patient-specific variables, and operator skill. Artifacts are distortions or errors in the elastographic image that can obscure or misrepresent tissue stiffness, potentially leading to misdiagnoses. Here, we'll explore key factors affecting image quality, common artifacts, and methods to mitigate these issues in ultrasound elastography.

4.1 Factors affecting image quality in elastography

The quality of elastography images is influenced by various technical and physiological factors:

a. Imaging technique (Strain vs. Shear wave elastography)

- Strain elastography (SE): Image quality is heavily dependent on the operator's ability to apply consistent compression or utilize natural motion (e.g., heartbeat). Uneven compression or excessive force can degrade image quality and lead to artifacts. The quality of the elastogram may also vary with tissue heterogeneity.

- Shear wave elastography (SWE): SWE tends to produce higher-quality images with less operator dependency, as it relies on acoustic radiation force to generate shear waves. However, SWE is sensitive to the depth of the region of interest (ROI), and its image quality decreases with increasing depth or excessive tissue attenuation (e.g., in obese patients).

b. Signal-to-noise ratio (SNR)

- SNR is crucial for high-quality elastograms. High SNR ensures that tissue displacements or shear wave propagation are accurately captured. Poor SNR can result in incomplete or inaccurate stiffness measurements.

- SNR is affected by factors such as acoustic attenuation in deeper tissues, the frequency of the ultrasound probe, and the presence of physiological noise (e.g., patient motion).

c. Tissue heterogeneity

- In heterogeneous tissues (e.g., tissues with fibrosis, fat, or calcifications), the elastic properties can vary greatly. This variability can affect both strain and shear wave elastography, leading to inconsistent stiffness measurements and degraded image quality.

d. Depth of the ROI

- Deeper tissues are harder to image with elastography due to increased attenuation of both the ultrasound and shear waves. This can result in reduced image quality and the potential for artifacts, particularly in abdominal imaging (e.g., liver elastography in obese patients).

- In SWE, the penetration depth depends on the frequency of the ultrasound probe. Lower frequencies allow greater depth penetration but at the expense of spatial resolution.

e. Transducer frequency

- Higher-frequency transducers provide better spatial resolution but have limited penetration depth. For superficial structures like thyroid or breast, high-frequency transducers are ideal. However, for deeper structures such as liver or kidneys, lower-frequency transducers are used, which may reduce image quality.

f. Motion artifacts

- Patient movement, such as breathing or heartbeats, can degrade elastography images, particularly in organs like the liver. Breath-hold techniques are often employed to minimize motion artifacts during liver elastography.

4.2 Common artifacts and mitigation in ultrasound elastography

Artifacts in elastography can misrepresent tissue stiffness, either artificially increasing or decreasing the measured values. The most common artifacts include:

a. Shadowing artifact

- Shadowing occurs when highly attenuating structures (e.g., bones, calcifications, or gas) block the ultrasound signal. This results in a loss of information in the shadowed area, leading to underestimation or lack of stiffness measurement (**Figure 7B**).

- Shear wave shadowing: In SWE, if the shear wave is blocked by a dense structure like a rib, it cannot propagate to deeper tissues, causing artifacts in the elastogram.

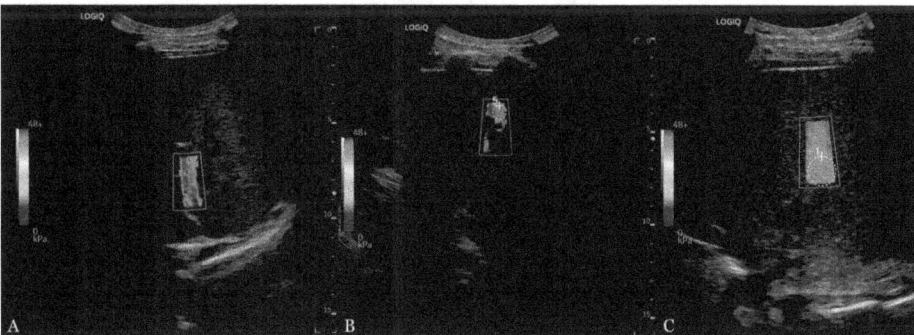

Figure 7.
Erroneous elastography values in a normal liver from artifact or user error at a GE LOGIQ 10 system. (A) Vertical bands across the ROI from motion with highly variable stiffness (3-48 kPa). (B) Artifactual liver stiffness acquired by placing ROI in a rib shadow. (C) Liver stiffness increased by 3.3 kPa in a normal liver by acquiring samples during maximum inspiration approximately 1 hour postprandial.

- Prevention: Adjusting the transducer position to avoid highly attenuating structures or changing the imaging window can reduce shadowing.

b. Reverberation artifact

- Reverberation occurs when the ultrasound signal bounces between two highly reflective surfaces, causing multiple echoes and resulting in false stiffness values.

- This artifact is common near superficial structures and can interfere with both strain and shear wave elastography by distorting tissue displacement measurements.

- Prevention: Adjusting the transducer angle or repositioning the transducer to minimize reverberations can help.

c. Compression artifact (in strain elastography)

- In strain elastography, uneven or excessive compression by the operator can lead to artifacts, particularly near the surface of the tissue. Over-compression can artificially increase the strain, making tissues appear softer than they are.

- Prevention: Proper training and practice in applying consistent, light compression can help reduce this artifact. Automatic compression techniques or external vibration sources can also be used to standardize compression.

d. Noise artifact

- A low SNR results in grainy or noisy elastograms, where the tissue stiffness is not clearly visualized. This can lead to false positives or false negatives in detecting tissue abnormalities, especially in SWE.

- Prevention: Improving the SNR by adjusting gain settings, using appropriate transducer frequency, and ensuring proper contact between the transducer and skin can help mitigate this artifact.

e. Side lobe artifact

- Side lobe artifacts occur when ultrasound energy from side lobes (off-axis beams) interferes with the main ultrasound signal, leading to incorrect elastography readings.

- These artifacts can be particularly problematic in SWE because side lobe energy can affect the generation and detection of shear waves.

- Prevention: Using high-quality transducers with good beamforming capabilities and adjusting the gain and focal zone settings can help reduce side lobe artifacts.

f. Inhomogeneity artifacts

- Tissue inhomogeneities such as reticular or confluent liver fibrosis, fat deposits, or necrotic masses can cause the shear wave to propagate unevenly, resulting in false stiffness measurements.

- In liver elastography, severe fatty liver disease (steatosis) can attenuate the shear wave, leading to underestimation of stiffness in deeper parts of the liver. However, lesser degrees of steatosis will actually reduce hepatic stiffness, masking the severity liver fibrosis.

- Prevention: Selecting ROIs that avoid areas of heterogeneity or using software algorithms to compensate for inhomogeneities can improve accuracy.

g. Edge artifact

- This artifact occurs near the borders of structures with large differences in stiffness. For example, the border of a stiff tumor and softer surrounding tissue can produce an artifact where the stiffness gradient is exaggerated or inaccurate.

- Prevention: Adjusting the ROI to exclude the very edge of structures can minimize the impact of edge artifacts.

h. Motion artifacts

- Both patient movement and internal motion (e.g., breathing, heartbeats) can interfere with shear wave propagation, leading to false readings.

- Visually this often manifests as vertical bands across the color map (**Figure 7A**).

- Prevention: Instructing the patient to hold their breath during imaging or using gating techniques (e.g., ECG synchronization for cardiac elastography) can reduce motion artifacts.

5. Bioeffect and safety of ultrasound elastography

Ultrasound elastography operates under certain physical principles that raise questions about its bioeffects and safety [27, 28]. Understanding these aspects is critical to ensure that elastography remains a safe modality for routine clinical use. This involves considering potential biological effects such as thermal and mechanical risks, as well as safety guidelines established by regulatory bodies.

5.1 Mechanisms of potential bioeffects

There are two primary mechanisms by which ultrasound, including that used in elastography, could potentially cause biological effects:

5.1.1 Thermal effects

- Ultrasound energy can cause tissue heating, particularly at higher intensities. This is referred to as the thermal index (TI), a measure of the potential temperature rise in tissue caused by ultrasound [9].

- During elastography, SWE uses focused acoustic radiation forces to generate shear waves. This requires a higher intensity compared to conventional B-mode imaging, and while it increases the risk of thermal effects, SWE is typically applied in short bursts (milliseconds), minimizing significant heating.

- SE relies on external compression or natural tissue movements, which do not generate heat, making it safer from a thermal perspective compared to SWE.

5.1.2 Mechanical effects

- Mechanical effects include non-thermal interactions like cavitation (the formation of bubbles in a liquid) or tissue displacement due to mechanical forces. These are quantified by the mechanical index (MI), which reflects the potential for cavitation or other mechanical bioeffects [9].

- In elastography, the application of acoustic radiation forces in SE and SWE can displace tissue, but the duration and energy of these forces are controlled to be within safe limits. For SE which uses external compression, it does not involve high-energy mechanical forces and thus carries lower mechanical risks.

- Cavitation is not typically a concern in elastography because the energy levels are well below the threshold required for the formation of gas bubbles in tissues.

5.2 Safety guidelines

Although ultrasound elastography is generally considered a safe, non-invasive imaging technique used to measure tissue stiffness, to ensure its safe and effective use, certain safety guidelines still should be followed. Several organizations such as FDA (Food and Drug Administration), AIUM (American Institute of Ultrasound in Medicine), and EFSUMB (European Federation of Societies for Ultrasound in Medicine and Biology) have established safety guidelines for the use of ultrasound elastography. Below are the key safety guidelines:

a. Minimize acoustic output: By following ALARA rule (As Low As Reasonably Achievable), the lowest acoustic output (TI and MI) that still provides adequate information should be used to minimize potential thermal and mechanical bioeffects on tissue. A TI of less than 1 is considered safe for most clinical applications and an MI below 1.9 is generally considered safe [29, 30].

b. Appropriate use of compression: When performing strain elastography with manual compression, care must be taken to avoid applying excessive force with the ultrasound probe as it could cause discomfort or injury to the patient. Excessive pressure can also distort measurements. Operators should be trained and certified in both standard and elastography techniques.

c. Sensitive organs: Care should be taken to avoid too much acoustic output over sensitive areas such as eyes, testes, and open wounds, or during long procedures to prevent tissue damage or burn.

d. Vulnerable patients: For pediatric, pregnant, elderly patients, or patients with conditions like osteoporosis, bone fractures, or severe skin conditions, extra care should be taken to avoid excessive transducer pressure.

e. Contraindications and precautions: Elastography may not be suitable for patients with severe inflammation or large volume abdominal ascites, where stiffness measurements may not reflect actual tissue stiffness.

6. Quality assurance of ultrasound elastography

Quality assurance (QA) in ultrasound elastography is essential to ensure that the technique produces reliable, consistent, and accurate measurements of tissue stiffness across different patients, operators, and systems. Here are the key components of quality assurance in ultrasound elastography.

6.1 Machine calibration and performance testing

To ensure that the ultrasound elastography system operates correctly and provides accurate stiffness measurements, routine calibration and performance testing are critical. This includes:

a. Phantom testing: Regular testing of ultrasound elastography systems using tissue-mimicking phantoms with known mechanical properties (e.g., known stiffness in kPa or shear wave velocity in m/s). Phantoms should simulate the physical properties of soft tissues and help verify the accuracy of elastography measurements.

  • Phantom types: Elastic and viscoelastic phantoms, which simulate different tissues, should be used to test both strain and shear wave elastography systems. These phantoms often have regions of varying stiffness, allowing the system to be tested for sensitivity and accuracy across a range of stiffness values. For example, Sun Nuclear Inc. provided two elasticity phantom models (model 046 and 039) for ultrasound elastography QA/QC (www. sunnuclear.com/ products/zerdine-ultrasound-phantom).

  • Accuracy verification: Measurements obtained from the ultrasound elastography system should closely match the known stiffness values of the phantom. Discrepancies between actual and expected values may indicate calibration issues, requiring adjustments to the system.

b. Reproducibility testing: Reproducibility of elastography measurements is critical. Multiple measurements on the same phantom should yield consistent results to ensure the system's reliability. The coefficient of variation (CV) should be low, typically under 10%, for good reproducibility [31].

c. System maintenance: Routine maintenance should be performed to ensure that the ultrasound system, transducer, and software components are functioning properly. Software updates may also include improvements to elastography algorithms, enhancing accuracy.

6.2 Standardization of acquisition protocols

Variability in ultrasound elastography measurements can occur due to differences in how the technique is applied, particularly in strain-based methods where manual compression is involved. To minimize variability, standardized acquisition protocols should be followed [10, 31, 32]:

a. Operator training: Operators should be well-trained in both the physics of elastography and the specific technique to ensure consistency. In the case of strain elastography, proper compression technique is critical for reliable results. For shear wave elastography, correct transducer placement and pressure are also essential.

b. Uniform compression/force: In strain elastography, ensuring uniform compression of the tissue is critical for reproducibility. Too much or too little pressure can affect the elastogram's accuracy. Acoustic radiation force used in shear wave elastography should also be consistent across measurements.

c. Patient positioning: Proper patient positioning and immobilization are crucial for reducing motion artifacts and ensuring consistent measurements. For example, during liver elastography, the patient should hold their breath to minimize motion artifacts from respiration.

d. Consistent region of interest (ROI): The ROI in elastography imaging should be consistently selected across measurements. ROIs should be placed in areas free of large blood vessels, calcifications, or other heterogeneities to avoid measurement errors.

e. Number of measurements: To improve accuracy, multiple elastography measurements (usually 5, 10 or more) should be acquired, and the median value of these measurements should be used to assess tissue stiffness. The spread (interquartile range, IQR) of the measurements can indicate variability and serve as a quality indicator.

f. Quality metrics: Many elastography systems provide real-time quality metrics (such as the shear wave quality map or the IQR/median ratio) that indicate the reliability of the current measurement. These metrics should be monitored to ensure that only high-quality data is included in the final assessment.

6.3 Intra-operator and inter-operator variability

a. Intra-Operator Variability: Variability within the same operator's measurements should be minimized by:

- Consistent application of the technique, using the same amount of force, ROI placement, and measurement protocols.

- Reproducibility tests should be performed regularly to monitor the consistency of an operator's measurements over time.

b. Inter-Operator Variability: Differences between operators can introduce variability in elastography measurements, especially in techniques like strain elastography that involve manual compression. To minimize this variability:

- Operators should undergo standardized training and certification processes to ensure consistency across different situations.

- Regular proficiency assessments should be conducted to ensure that operators adhere to best practices.

6.4 Patient-specific factors

Patient-specific factors can influence elastography measurements. QA protocols must take these factors into account:

a. Body mass index (BMI) and Subcutaneous Fat: In patients with high BMI or large amounts of subcutaneous fat, shear waves may not propagate effectively, leading to inaccurate measurements, particularly in deeper tissues like the liver. Techniques such as adjusting the frequency of the ultrasound probe, using different transducers, or modifying the measurement depth can help address these issues.

b. Breath holding and motion artifacts: For liver elastography, patients are usually asked to hold their breath during measurements to avoid motion artifacts from respiration. Ensuring proper patient cooperation is essential for obtaining reliable data.

c. Tissue heterogeneity: Tissues with heterogeneities, such as fibrosis, calcifications, or fatty infiltration, may affect the accuracy of elastography measurements. The operator should be trained to avoid regions with such heterogeneities or adjust measurement protocols accordingly.

6.5 Regulatory standards and guidelines

International and national guidelines for elastography quality assurance are essential for maintaining high standards in clinical practice. For example, EFSUMB provides guidelines for the use of elastography, including equipment calibration, operator training, and clinical protocols for different elastography techniques [32]. The AIUM provides recommendations for ultrasound elastography, emphasizing quality control measures, training, and equipment maintenance [33]. Radiology Society of North America (RSNA) Quantitative Imaging Biomarker Alliance (QIBA) standardizes methods to create biomarkers that meet a claimed performance and publishes profiles and consensus of ultrasound elastography [3, 31, 34]. The World Federation for Ultrasound in Medicine and Biology (WFUMB) published a series of elastography guidelines in liver, breast, thyroid, and prostate [10].

7. Conclusion

Ultrasound elastography is a specialized technique that measures tissue stiffness by utilizing the principles of mechanical wave propagation within soft tissues.

The core physical principle involves the generation of strain or shear waves through tissue, where the displacement or velocity of these waves is directly related to tissue stiffness. The primary imaging techniques in ultrasound elastography include strain elastography and shear wave elastography. In response to excitation, strain elastography measures tissue displacement, whereas shear wave elastography quantifies shear wave speed. Elastograms with either qualitive or quantitative metrics are provided to assess abnormalities of tissue stiffness such as liver fibrosis, breast lesions, and thyroid nodules.

Image quality in ultrasound elastography can be influenced by several factors, including the uniformity of tissue compression, patient movement, and depth of the target tissue. Artifacts such as noise from surrounding tissues, attenuation at greater depths, or inaccuracies due to improper probe handling can degrade image quality. To address these challenges, careful technique, optimized equipment settings, and robust algorithms are employed to enhance image quality and reduce artifacts. Ultrasound elastography is considered safe due to the non-ionizing nature of ultrasound waves and low energy deposition. It is a repeatable and non-invasive procedure, making it well-suited for longitudinal monitoring. Quality assurance plays a vital role in ensuring accurate and reproducible results. This includes regular calibration of ultrasound machines, adherence to standardized imaging protocols, and continuous training for operators to maintain consistency in elastogram acquisition and interpretation.

Overall, ultrasound elastography with proper implementation and special consideration is a non-invasive, real-time, safe, reliable, and qualitive/quantitative technique which can be utilized to assess tissue stiffness in clinical and research applications.

Author details

Yonggang Lu* and Brian Di Giacinto
Department of Radiology, Medical College of Wisconsin, Milwaukee, USA

*Address all correspondence to: yolu@mcw.edu

IntechOpen

References

[1] Sigrist RMS, Liau J, Kaffas AE, Chammas MC, Willmann JK. Ultrasound elastography: Review of techniques and clinical applications. Theranostics. 2017;**7**(5):1303-1329. DOI: 10.7150/thno.18650

[2] Ozturk A, Grajo JR, Dhyani M, Anthony BW, Samir AE. Principles of ultrasound elastography. Abdominal Radiology. 2018;**43**(4):773-785. DOI: 10.1007/s00261-018-1475-6

[3] Barr RG, Wilson SR, Rubens D, Garcia-Tsao G, Ferraioli G. Update to the society of radiologists in ultrasound liver elastography consensus statement. Radiology. 2020;**296**(2):263-274. DOI: 10.1148/radiol.2020192437

[4] Barr RG, Zhang Z. Shear-wave elastography of the breast: Value of a quality measure and comparison with strain elastography. Radiology. 2015;**275**(1):45-53. DOI: 10.1148/radiol.14132404

[5] van Holsbeeck M, Soliman S, Van Kerkhove F, Craig J. Advanced musculoskeletal ultrasound techniques: What are the applications? AJR. American Journal of Roentgenology. 2021;**216**(2):436-445. DOI: 10.2214/AJR.20.22840

[6] Mederacke I, Wursthorn K, Kirschner J, et al. Food intake increases liver stiffness in patients with chronic or resolved hepatitis C virus infection. Liver International. 2009;**29**(10):1500-1506. DOI: 10.1111/j.1478-3231.2009.02100.x|

[7] Hedrick WR. Technology for Diagnostic Sonography. St. Louis: Elsevier Health Sciences; 2012

[8] Karam AR, Beland MD. Liver ultrasound elastography: Review of techniques and clinical applications. R.I. Medical Journal. 2013;**103**(5):26-29

[9] Bushberg JTS, Leidholdt EM, Boone JM. The Essential Physics of Medical Imaging. Philadelphia: Wolters Kluwer Health; 2020

[10] Shiina T, Nightingale KR, Palmeri ML, et al. WFUMB guidelines and recommendations for clinical use of ultrasound elastography: Part 1: Basic principles and terminology. Ultrasound in Medicine and Biology. 2015;**41**(5):1126-1147. DOI: 10.1016/j.ultrasmedbio.2015.03.009

[11] Ngo HH, Poulard T, Brum J, Gennisson JL. Anisotropy in ultrasound shear wave elastography: An add-on to muscles characterization. Frontiers in Physiology. 2022;**13**:1000612. DOI: 10.3389/fphys.2022.1000612

[12] Grenier N, Gennisson JL, Cornelis F, Le Bras Y, Couzi L. Renal ultrasound elastography. Diagnostic and Interventional Imaging. 2013;**94**(5):545-550. DOI: 10.1016/j.diii.2013.02.003

[13] Leong SS, Wong JHD, Md Shah MN, et al. Stiffness and anisotropy effect on shear wave elastography: A phantom and in vivo renal study. Ultrasound in Medicine and Biology. 2020;**46**(1):34-45. DOI: 10.1016/j.ultrasmedbio.2019.08.011

[14] Correia M, Deffieux T, Chatelin S, Provost J, Tanter M, Pernot M. 3D elastic tensor imaging in weakly transversely isotropic soft tissues. Physics in Medicine and Biology. 2018;**63**(15):155005. DOI: 10.1088/1361-6560/aacfaf

[15] Ozkan F, Menzilcioglu MS, Duymus M, Yildiz S. Accurate measurement of strain ratio in

quasi-static elastography. Polskie Archiwum Medycyny Wewnętrznej. 2014;**124**(10):556

[16] Ramalli A, Basset O, Cachard C, Boni E, Tortoli P. Frequency-domain-based strain estimation and high-frame-rate imaging for quasi-static elastography. IEEE Transactions on Ultrasonics, Ferroelectrics, and Frequency Control. 2012;**59**(4):817-824. DOI: 10.1109/TUFFC.2012.2260

[17] Mehanna H, Deeks JJ, Boelaert K, et al. Real-time ultrasound elastography in the diagnosis of newly identified thyroid nodules in adults: The ElaTION RCT. Health Technology Assessment. 2024;**28**(46):1-51. DOI: 10.3310/PLEQ4874

[18] Motosugi U, Ichikawa T, Niitsuma Y, Araki T. Acoustic radiation force impulse elastography of the liver: Can fat deposition in the liver affect the measurement of liver stiffness? Japanese Journal of Radiology. 2011;**29**(9):639-643. DOI: 10.1007/s11604-011-0607-5

[19] Lee SM, Kim MJ, Yoon JH, et al. Comparison of point and 2-dimensional shear wave elastography for the evaluation of liver fibrosis. Ultrasonography. 2020;**39**(3):288-297. DOI: 10.14366/usg.19090

[20] Deffieux T, Montaldo G, Tanter M, Fink M. Shear wave spectroscopy for in vivo quantification of human soft tissues visco-elasticity. IEEE Transactions on Medical Imaging. 2009;**28**(3):313-322. DOI: 10.1109/TMI.2008.925077

[21] Huang C, Song P, Mellema DC, et al. Three-dimensional shear wave elastography on conventional ultrasound scanners with external vibration. Physics in Medicine and Biology. 2020;**65**(21):215009. DOI: 10.1088/1361-6560/aba5ea

[22] Gennisson JL, Provost J, Deffieux T, et al. 4-D ultrafast shear-wave imaging. IEEE Transactions on Ultrasonics, Ferroelectrics, and Frequency Control. 2015;**62**(6):1059-1065. DOI: 10.1109/TUFFC.2014.006936

[23] Bhatt M, Yazdani L, Destrempes F, et al. Multiparametric in vivo ultrasound shear wave viscoelastography on farm-raised fatty duck livers: Human radiology imaging applied to food sciences. Poultry Science. 2021;**100**(6):101076. DOI: 10.1016/j.psj.2021.101076

[24] Foucher J, Chanteloup E, Vergniol J, et al. Diagnosis of cirrhosis by transient elastography (FibroScan): A prospective study. Gut. 2006;**55**(3):403-408. DOI: 10.1136/gut.2005.069153

[25] Chamming's F, Le-Frere-Belda MA, Latorre-Ossa H, et al. Supersonic shear wave elastography of response to anti-cancer therapy in a xenograft tumor model. Ultrasound in Medicine and Biology. 2016;**42**(4):924-930. DOI: 10.1016/j.ultrasmedbio.2015.12.001

[26] Tzschatzsch H, Ipek-Ugay S, Guo J, et al. In vivo time-harmonic multifrequency elastography of the human liver. Physics in Medicine and Biology. 2014;**59**(7):1641-1654. DOI: 10.1088/0031-9155/59/7/1641

[27] Izadifar Z, Babyn P, Chapman D. Mechanical and biological effects of ultrasound: A review of present knowledge. Ultrasound in Medicine and Biology. 2017;**43**(6):1085-1104. DOI: 10.1016/j.ultrasmedbio.2017.01.023

[28] Shankar H, Pagel PS. Potential adverse ultrasound-related biological effects: A critical review. Anesthesiology. 2011;**115**(5):1109-1124. DOI: 10.1097/ALN.0b013e31822fd1f1

[29] Butler S, Ashcroft K, Arrowsmith S, Griffiths R, Studd A.

Assessment of thermal index compliance in clinical ultrasound examinations. Ultrasound. 2024;**32**(3):151-156. DOI: 10.1177/1742271X231225057

[30] Meltzer RS. Food and drug administration ultrasound device regulation: The output display standard, the "mechanical index," and ultrasound safety. Journal of the American Society of Echocardiography. 1996;**9**(2):216-220. DOI: 10.1016/s0894-7317(96)90035-8|

[31] QIBA Profile: Ultrasound Measurement of Shear Wave Speed for Estimation of Liver Fibrosis. [Internet]. 2024. Available from: https://qibawiki. rsna.org

[32] Bamber J, Cosgrove D, Dietrich CF, et al. EFSUMB guidelines and recommendations on the clinical use of ultrasound elastography. Part 1: Basic principles and technology. Ultraschall in der Medizin. 2013;**34**(2):169-184. DOI: 10.1055/s-0033-1335205

[33] Elastography. [Internet]. 2024. Available from: https://www.aium.org/ practice-topics/elastography

[34] Palmeri ML, Milkowski A, Barr R, et al. Radiological Society of North America/quantitative imaging biomarker Alliance shear wave speed bias quantification in elastic and viscoelastic phantoms. Journal of Ultrasound in Medicine. 2021;**40**(3):569-581. DOI: 10.1002/jum.15609

Chapter 3

Ultrasound Elastographic Features of Focal Liver Lesions: A Review

Evren Üstüner, Kemal Altınbaş and Metin Yavuz

Abstract

The assessment of the mechanical properties of focal liver lesions (FLLs), such as stiffness, deformation, and elasticity, using liver sonoelastography remains an area of ongoing investigation. This review aims to summarize the current evidence on FLLs, highlighting the technical and methodological limitations of existing studies, as well as exploring potential future applications. It will cover essential factors for successful study execution, including the types and limitations of sonoelastographic methods, proper technique implementation to avoid common pitfalls, and guidance on constructing reports to convey critical information. Elastographic measurements are typically based on the assumption that malignant lesions are stiffer than benign ones, though variations in lesion structure and surrounding liver parenchyma may affect the results. Although the accuracy of elastography for FLLs is not ideal and does not always provide perfect differentiation, it can serve as a useful adjunct in patients unable to undergo contrast-enhanced computed tomography (CT) or magnetic resonance imaging (MRI) or in combination with other sonographic techniques such as multiparametric ultrasound. It may also help differentiate between types of FLLs when the differential diagnosis is narrowed to specific subgroups. Additionally, elastographic techniques can assist in biopsy guidance and in evaluating treatment responses to ablative therapies. The integration of artificial intelligence-assisted technologies may further enhance the diagnostic potential of elastography for FLLs in the future.

Keywords: ultrasound, elastography, focal liver lesions, liver mass, hemangioma, hepatocellular carcinoma, cholangiocarcinoma

1. Introduction

Noninvasive diagnosis of focal liver lesions (FLLs) aims to differentiate benign from malignant lesions. Multimodal approaches combining ultrasound, contrast-enhanced computed tomography (CT), magnetic resonance imaging (MRI), positron emission tomography-computed tomography (PET-CT), and biopsy are tailored to individual patient characteristics, considering factors like safety, contraindications, costs, and availability [1, 2]. Ultrasound (US) is widely used for its accessibility and cost-effectiveness, but its sensitivity varies (40–80%) depending on lesion size, location, echogenicity, and operator expertise, with challenges in detecting small lesions (<1 cm) or those in cirrhotic livers [3, 4]. To improve accuracy, advanced, multiparametric ultrasound techniques, such as contrast-enhanced ultrasound (CEUS) and shear wave elastography

(SWE), are employed. CEUS, with a sensitivity of 92% and specificity of 87–90%, rivals CT and MRI [1–6]. For instance, CEUS achieved a sensitivity of 92.9% and specificity of 89.7% in detecting malignant lesions in a 2014 study by Zhang et al. [7].

Elastography techniques assess tissue stiffness and viscosity, with malignant lesions being stiffer due to factors like extracellular matrix (ECM) changes, desmoplasia, and interstitial pressure. ECM stiffness significantly impacts tumor morphology, aggressiveness, and treatment response, while benign lesions are often encapsulated with minimal ECM changes [8, 9]. SWE lacks sufficient sensitivity and specificity for routine FLL differentiation. European Federation of Societies for Ultrasound in Medicine and Biology (EFSUMB) and World Federation for Ultrasound in Medicine and Biology (WFUMB) consider SWE investigational, citing variability in lesion composition, imaging methods, and patient factors [10–13]. A multiparametric approach incorporating clinical context, B-mode imaging, CEUS, SWE, and Doppler techniques is recommended for optimal FLL evaluation [1, 2, 6].

2. Types of elastography used in assessment of FLLs

Strain elastography (SE) qualitatively assesses tissue stiffness through external compressive forces, making it suitable for superficial structures. However, SE is operator-dependent, has low resolution, and results may vary due to inconsistent wave dissipation [6, 15, 16]. Real-time SE provides elasticity maps and semi-quantitative measures like strain ratio and hardness percentage, often relying on color-coded scales [14–17]. For instance, the Elasticity Type of Liver Tumor (ETLT) system categorizes strain patterns into four levels (A to D) based on stiffness, as described by Kato et al., later expanded into modified ETLT [16, 17].

Dynamic methods like transient elastography (TE) and acoustic radiation force impulse (ARFI) provide quantitative stiffness assessment by analyzing shear wave propagation. TE (one dimensional SWE (1D-SWE)), commonly used for liver fibrosis assessment, lacks B-mode imaging and is unsuitable for FLLs [14, 15]. ARFI enables localized tissue stiffness evaluation through virtual touch imaging (VTI) and point shear wave elastography (pSWE), integrating B-mode imaging and offering both semi and absolute quantitative analysis using a fixed 1 cc or 5-6x10 cm region of interest (ROI). Technology relies on a brief acoustic trigger pulse that generates lateral shear waves quantified by Doppler (ElastPQ) or radiofrequency echo-based tracking [4, 6, 10, 14, 15]. ARFI measurements, though effective up to 8 cm, are influenced by factors like breathing and motion artifacts [14, 15, 18].

Two-dimensional SWE (2D-SWE) uses focused ARFI pulses for high-resolution stiffness maps, enabling both qualitative and quantitative assessments of FLLs. It provides real-time color-coded stiffness visualization and higher spatial resolution than ARFI or TE. However, inter-vendor variability and depth-related limitations impact its consistency, emphasizing the need for standardization [18–20]. Color scales, set by the vendor, typically range from blue/green (low stiffness) to red (high stiffness). SWE measures stiffness as shear wave velocity (m/s) or as Young's modulus (kPa), calculated using tissue density and shear wave speed that are convertible based on the formula $E = 3\rho c2$ where E represents elasticity, c is the shear wave speed and ρ is the tissue density, often approximated as that of water. pSWE measurements are often expressed using meter per second (m/s) and 2D-SWE measurements as kiloPascals (kPa) [1, 10, 14, 15, 18–20]. Three Dimensional SWE (3D-SWE) offers volumetric analysis but is time-intensive and prone to motion artifacts [21].

In 2D-SWE, each system has defined upper and lower limits within its color spectrum. For instance, the Aixplorer system (Supersonic Imagine, France) has an upper color spectrum limit of 70 kPa [4, 45]. Similarly, with ARFI Virtual Touch Quantification (VTQ), the Siemens Acuson S2000 device (Siemens, California) could not reliably quantify lesions with VTQ values below 0.5 m/s or above 4.4–5 m/s [29, 36]. Stiffness values derived from deformation and strain are influenced by the differences in frequency of excitative ARFI pulses, technology, calibration and algorithms which may vary by 10–12% among manufacturers. Consequently, it is essential to be aware to this inter-vendor variability and use the same device or technology for consistent comparison or follow-up evaluations of stiffness in specific tissues and refer to established cross system comparison manuals when interpreting results [10, 15, 16, 18].

Studies comparing methods show similar diagnostic performance. For example, Nacheva-Georgieva et al. found pSWE and 2D-SWE equally effective in differentiating benign from malignant lesions, with AUROCs of 100% [20]. Hu et al.'s meta-analysis reported comparable sensitivity and specificity for pSWE (82% sensitivity, 82% specificity) and 2D-SWE (84% sensitivity, 82% specificity) [22]. Sporea et al. found that both VTQ and ElastPQ are effective in gauging liver stiffness; however, ElastPQ consistently yielded lower values than VTQ, a discrepancy they attributed to the differing physical principles of each technique [18]. Despite advancements, limitations like depth related shear wave attenuation, mechanical constraints, and inter-vendor differences necessitate cautious interpretation and ongoing technological improvements [6, 15].

3. Technique

Adhering to WFUMB, Society of Radiologists in Ultrasound (SRU), and EFSUMB guidelines ensures consistency and minimizes variability in elastography assessments. However, not all FLLs are suitable for elastographic evaluation. Hu et al. in their metanalysis, reported that measurement infeasibility was observed in 1.2 to 26.3% of cases, with an average rate of 12.7% due to technical and patient-related factors like lesion depth, motion artifacts, and poor acoustic windows [22]. Despite these limitations, optimized techniques and equipment, such as fasting, proper positioning, and selecting the best acoustic window, can improve success rates to over 90% [11, 22–24].

SWE measurements depend on lesion depth, location, and liver conditions. Depth-related attenuation and artifacts complicate measurements in lesions >8 cm deep or in left liver segments affected by cardiac motion [10, 11, 25]. The ROI measurements should be done in suspended breathing on homogeneous, peripheral, stiff areas, avoiding necrotic, central, calcified, marginal regions and should avoid the liver capsule and large vessels [10, 24–27]. Naganuma et al. recommend placing the ROI away from the liver capsule to avoid reverberation artifacts and refraining from positioning it posterior to lesions to minimize refraction and reflection issues at tissue interfaces. They also suggest selecting the least irregular hepatic surface for measurements in cirrhotic livers and reducing probe compression when performing 2D-SWE [19]. If more than one lesion is present, most representative and easiest to measure is chosen and if lesion's size is more than 3 cm and heterogenous, multiple large ROI can be used to cover the lesion and measurements are averaged [28]. Color maps can be used to guide the ROIs to the stiffest parts of the lesion [24]. Guibal et al. found no correlation between lesion size and mean stiffness in both benign and malignant FLLs using 2D-SWE, emphasizing that elastometry of FLLs is unique to the lesion [29].

The stiffness of surrounding liver parenchyma can influence the accuracy of SWE of FLLs, particularly in cirrhosis, steatosis, or after oncological treatments [15, 30, 31]. Frulio et al. examined the stiffness of surrounding liver tissue in relation to FLLs and found that increased parenchymal shear wave velocity (SWV) values were not limited to fibrosis but were also observed in cases of steatosis, chemotherapy, peliosis, congestion, portal embolization, and portal thrombosis. Interestingly, they noted that, in some patients, elevated SWV values were recorded in normal liver tissue without any apparent reason [30]. The study by Hwang et al. on liver phantoms using 2D-SWE demonstrated that stiffness values of phantoms were influenced by both the background stiffness and the depth of inclusions. Stiffness of lesion phantoms was significantly higher in cirrhotic simulations compared to normal (13.9 vs. 10.2 kPa), and higher variability and less reliability were noted at 7 cm depths compared to 3–5 cm depths and lesion conspicuity decreased significantly in lesions less than 1 cm [32]. Some studies suggest using relative stiffness metrics (lesion-to-liver ratio) to enhance diagnostic accuracy, though results vary [30, 33–37]. Summing or comparing stiffness values between lesions and adjacent tissue shows potential in improving malignancy differentiation [24, 35, 36].

Reproducibility of SWE measurements is generally high, with strong intra- and interobserver agreement, particularly for shallow, homogeneous lesions [24, 25, 32, 35]. Elastography values often vary within and among tumors due to differences in internal composition, with heterogeneity more common in larger, necrotic malignant tumors, potentially indicating malignancy [28, 30]. Metrics such as an interquartile range (IQR)-to-median ratio > 0.3 in ARFI and a standard deviation (SD) >5 kPa in 2D-SWE suggest heterogeneity [29, 30, 38]. Larger ROIs increase SD and reduce mean elasticity (Emean) due to sampling varied elasticity areas, including necrotic regions. Smaller, fixed ROIs targeting stiff areas provide more precise results [24, 25]. Grgurevic found no significant difference between minimum, mean, and maximum elasticity (Emin, Emean, and Emax) for malignancy differentiation [28]. Gerber reported similar findings but noted sensitivity and specificity trade-offs depending on ROI placement, with Emax from the stiffest areas performing best [39, 40].

4. Reporting

When evaluating FLLs with elastography, it is crucial to document B-mode ultrasound features, including lesion location, size, shape, depth, echogenicity, and morphology. Precise localization using the Couinaud classification and noting whether lesions are incidental or associated with fibrosis, malignancy, or parenchymal changes (e.g., due to chemotherapy or radiation) are essential [39, 41]. The vascularity of lesions should be assessed, excluding aneurysms that mimic FLLs. For elastography, the rationale for lesion selection must be documented. In pSWE, the ROI placement site should be noted, while in 2D-SWE, both ROI size and placement must be specified. SWE measurements, typically median values from at least 3–5 ROIs up to 10, should be reported in Young's modulus (kPa) or shear wave velocity (m/s). Including maximum elasticity (Emax) and relative stiffness ratio (RR) can enhance diagnostic accuracy [21, 24, 40]. Adherence to quality parameters such as stability index (>90%) and IQR/m (<30%) is critical for reliable results, and these indicators should be documented [10–12]. Device variability (10–12%) necessitates using the same system for follow-ups, and the type of elastography, device, and probe should be recorded [10–12, 18]. Saving dynamic and still images in picture archiving and communication system (PACS) and ensuring post-processing capabilities are recommended. Awareness of confounding factors affecting stiffness values should be noted in reports to enhance diagnostic accuracy and management.

5. Methodological limitations of elastographic studies on FLLs

Elastography studies of FLLs face several limitations that affect reliability and generalizability. Many studies are retrospective or case series without assessing inter- and intra-observer variability, and small, homogeneous sample sizes often lack diversity in tumor subtypes [6, 28, 43, 44]. Benign lesions like hemangiomas (HHs) and focal nodular hyperplasias (FNHs) are well-represented, whereas rarer subtypes, such as cirrhotic nodules (CNs) and hepatocellular adenomas (HAs), are underrepresented. Similarly, malignant lesions such as cholangiocarcinomas (CCCs), lymphomas, and sarcomas are less frequently studied, reducing statistical power [33, 45]. Most studies diagnose FLLs based on imaging (CT, MRI, CEUS) rather than histopathology, potentially misidentifying subtypes, as tumor stiffness values vary with histological composition [25, 28, 46]. Tumor heterogeneity, both inter- and intra-lesional, further influences outcomes, particularly in metastatic lesions from diverse origins. Indicators like increased IQR/m or standard deviation may reflect this variability [29, 30, 38].

Inconsistencies in shear wave elastography (SWE) methods, such as ROI size and placement, further challenge comparisons. Lesions <10 mm are often excluded, and studies differ in ROI placement—whether targeting the stiffest part, the entire lesion, or averaging areas [28, 39, 40, 42, 47]. The number of measurements also varies, with studies using two to ten measurements, and approaches to surrounding parenchyma assessment differ [28, 30, 33, 48]. Absolute stiffness values, relative ratios, or sums are inconsistently applied [24, 33–35]. Variations in SWE technologies, including ARFI, pSWE, and 2D-SWE, add to study heterogeneity, complicating cross-study comparisons and interpretation [10, 14, 18].

6. General elastographic evaluation of focal liver lesions

Differentiating benign from malignant FLLs is critical for timely management. While most FLLs are benign and incidental, primary liver cancer is the sixth most common cancer and the fourth leading cause of cancer-related deaths globally [49]. Common benign lesions include HHs, FNHs, and hepatocellular adenomas (HAs), whereas metastases and hepatocellular carcinoma (HCCs) are the most common malignant lesions [41, 49]. Initial evaluation involves B-mode and Color Doppler ultrasound (CDUS) to exclude cystic and vascular lesions and assess the background liver parenchyma [28, 41]. Factors such as old age, male gender, anemia, elevated alpha-fetoprotein, and liver fibrosis increase the likelihood of malignancy [41, 50].

SWE differentiates lesions based on stiffness, with malignant lesions generally stiffer than benign ones. CCCs, metastases, and HCCs are among the stiffest, while HHs and HAs are the softest, though stiffness values often overlap [27, 29, 30, 33, 48, 51]. HCCs in cirrhotic livers may appear softer due to the stiff background, complicating differentiation [25, 27, 29, 52]. Techniques like histogram analysis of elasticity maps may improve diagnostic accuracy by identifying patterns unique to benign or malignant lesions [53, 54].

Stiffness values can also reflect tumor aggression and therapy response. For example, HCCs with stiffness >19.53 kPa are associated with poor outcomes with programmed cell death protein 1 (PD-1) inhibitors, while increased liver stiffness correlates with reduced responses to sorafenib [55, 56]. Peritumoral stiffness often increases due to tumor invasion and ECM remodeling, though its diagnostic accuracy remains moderate compared to paratumoral measurements (>2 cm from the lesion) [57]. Matrix stiffness directly influences tumor progression and resistance to treatment. Studies show HCC cells in stiffer environments exhibit higher proliferation and dedifferentiation, emphasizing stiffness as a marker for malignancy and treatment planning [8, 9, 55, 56]. Further research is needed to refine elastography's role in clinical decision-making **Table 1**.

7. Elastographic studies in differentiation of malignant from benign lesions

Strain elastography (SE) has been utilized with histogram and hardness percentage analyses for FLL evaluation. Kato et al. achieved 92.7% diagnostic accuracy in intraoperative SE, showing HCCs as softer (pattern B) and metastases as stiffer (pattern D) on a four-tier ETLT color map [16]. Sandulescu et al. achieved 92.5% sensitivity and 88.6% accuracy using SE histogram analysis [53], while Gheorghe et al. found blue-coded stiffness and hypervascularity as key indicators for HCC, with a blue intensity cut-off value of 128.9 yielding an area under the curve (AUROC) of 0.94 [54]. Cesario et al. reported that modified ETLT improved benign-malignant differentiation but with reduced accuracy. A strain ratio cut-off of 1.2 provided 90.9% sensitivity and 87.5% specificity [58]. Abdel-Latif et al. [59], Guibal et al. [29], and Park et al. demonstrated 2D-SWE color maps as effective tools for differentiation [25]. Frulio et al. and Abdel-Latif et al. highlighted that FNHs can mimic malignancies on SE [30, 59]. The discrepancies between color maps and stiffness values stem from the qualitative nature of SE versus ARFI technology, which measures strain via shear wave propagation [14].

Early studies focused on ARFI pSWE, while 2D-SWE gained prominence after 2015. Malignant lesions generally show higher stiffness than benign ones, but overlapping SWE values limit diagnostic accuracy. SWV cut-offs range from 1.5–2.7 m/s (ARFI) and 22.3–39.6 kPa (2D-SWE). The sensitivity and specificity for differentiating benign from malignant lesions using elastography cut-offs range from 66 to 93% and 30 to 95%, respectively, with AUROCs between 0.70 and 0.99 (6.22,51,60–63). CCCs generally have the highest stiffness, followed by metastases and HCCs, though some HCCs appear softer due to tissue composition and necrosis. Subtype differentiation is weaker in studies with fewer metastatic or CCC cases [6, 22, 51, 60–63]. Ying et al.'s meta-analysis of ARFI elastography (590 lesions) reported a sensitivity of 86% and specificity of 89%, with a hierarchical summary ROC of 0.94 [61]. Ma et al., analyzing six studies (448 lesions), found a sensitivity of 85% and specificity of 84%

Benign liver lesion	Stiffness	Malignant liver lesion	Stiffness
Hemangioma	Low to moderate	HCC	Low to high
Focal nodular hyperplasia	Moderate to high	Metastatic lesions	Moderate to very high
Hepatocellular adenomas	Low to moderate	Cholangiocarcinoma	Moderate to very high
Regenerative nodules	Moderate to high		
Dysplastic nodules	Moderate to very high		

Table 1.
Stiffness of common benign and malignant lesions.

Study (meta-analysis)	year	Number of lesions	No. of studies	Elastography technology	SWE value cut-off (Emean)	Sensitivity	Specificity	HSROC
Ying et al. [14]	2012	590	8	ARFI	1.5–2.7 m/s	86% (95%CI:0.74–0.93)	89% (95%CI:0.81–0.94)	0.94 (95%CI:0.91–0.96)
Ma et al. [71]	2014	448	4 + 2	ARFI + SE	1.56 m/s	85% (95%CI:0.80–0.89)	84% (95%CI:0.80–0.88)	0.9328
Jiao et al. [72]	2017	1046	8 + 1	ARFI+2D-SWE	1.8–2.73 m/s 13 kPa	82.2% (95%CI:0.73.4–0.88.5)	80,2% (95%CI:0.73.3–0.85.7)	0.87 (95%CI:0.84–0.90)
Hu et al. [39]	2019	1894	12 + 3	ARFI+2D-SWE	1,.8–2.5 m/s 20.7–24.43 kPa	82% (95%CI:0.77–0.86)	82% (95%CI:0.76–0.87)	0.89 (95%CI:0.86–0.91)

SE: strain elastography. HSROC: hierarchial summary receiver operating characteristics.

Table 2.
Overall summary of meta-analysis studies related to shear wave elastography cut-off value, sensitivity, specificity, and accuracy related to differentiation of malignant and benign focal liver lesions are presented.

using a 1.56 m/s SWV cut-off, achieving an AUROC of 0.933 [62]. Jiao et al. reviewed nine studies (1046 lesions), reporting a sensitivity of 82.2%, specificity of 80.2%, and summary ROC of 0.87 [63]. Similarly, Hu et al., in a review of 15 studies (1894 lesions), reported a sensitivity and specificity of 82%, with a summary ROC of 0.89 using SWV cut-offs of 1.82–2.5 m/s (**Table 2**) [22].

Maximal elasticity (Emax) has shown advantages over Emean and Emin values in differentiating FLLs. Zhang et al. found that Emax values (cut-off 1.945 m/s) achieved an AUROC of 0.978, with sensitivity and specificity of 92.9 and 91.7%, respectively [42]. Tian et al. reported that Emax improved specificity (83.7 vs. 72%) compared to Emean but slightly reduced sensitivity (87.7 vs. 90.2%) [24]. Guo et al. observed moderate diagnostic accuracy for Emax with an AUROC of 0.74, while Grgurevic found no significant differences among Emax, Emean, and Emin [28, 40].

Combining SWE with other sonographic modalities, such as CEUS, improves diagnostic accuracy. Singla et al. reported that SWE combined with B-mode imaging increased predictive accuracy from 66 to 91.4% [46]. Zhang et al. found CEUS and SWE together achieved 96.4% accuracy compared to 91.8% for CEUS alone [7]. Ruan et al. reported increased specificity and AUROC when adding SWE to CEUS for benign lesion diagnosis, while SWE alone showed a 100% NPV for benign lesions and PPV for malignant lesions at specific stiffness thresholds [64]. Grgurevic et al. introduced a malignancy score combining SWE metrics that included lesion stiffness, relative stiffness and stiffness variance, achieving 96% accuracy [28]. In the study by Wu et al. when VTQ was combined with CEUS, the results improved compared to VTQ alone but did not improve significantly compared to CEUS alone [51, 65]. Da Silva et al. highlighted that SWE enhanced CEUS by improving specificity and identifying challenging lesions [66]. These studies suggest that SWE complements CEUS by reducing false positives and improving diagnostic performance in complex cases.

Elastography values often vary in large or necrotic tumors, indicating malignancy. High intralesional stiffness variation, such as an IQR-to-mean ratio ≥ 0.3 or elasticity SD ≥ 5 kPa, correlates with malignancy [29]. Grgurevic et al. found significant stiffness variability with an AUROC of 0.62, while Tian et al. reported an AUROC of 0.915 using an elasticity SD (E-SD) cut-off of 5.50 kPa, achieving 82.35% sensitivity and 89.8% specificity [24, 28] Guibal et al. noted that while malignant lesions like metastases showed greater heterogeneity, benign lesions such as focal nodular hyperplasia (FNH) could also exhibit variability (**Table 3**) [29].

8. Contribution of background liver stiffness measurements to benign and malignant FLLs differentiation

pSWE and 2D-SWE target lesion stiffness, but adding surrounding liver stiffness or relative elasticity ratio (RR) offers limited diagnostic improvement [24, 25, 30, 51, 67, 68]. Most studies found liver stiffness higher in HCC patients compared to the background liver [27, 39, 52]. Ronot et al. noted no significant RR changes in liver steatosis, with FLLs consistently stiffer in normal livers (26.8 ± 14 vs. 8.2 ± 3.1 kPa) [45]. Heide et al. found no significant stiffness difference between benign and malignant lesions without cirrhosis (1.47 ± 1.08 vs. 1.57 ± 1.51 m/s) [33]. Frulio et al. observed higher liver stiffness in malignancy but noted overlap among the lesions [30]. Park et al. reported lower stiffness for HCC (45.72 ± 35.65 kPa) compared to metastases (67.43 ± 43.39 kPa) but higher than benign lesions (22.05 ± 17.24 kPa); RR differences were not significant [25].

Study	Year	Number of lesions	Type of elastography –vendor	SWE value cut-off	Sensitivity	Specificity
Cho et al. [44]*	2010	60	ARFI – Acuson S2000-Siemens	2 m/s	74%	82%
Davies et al. [23]**	2011	45	ARFI – Acuson S2000-Siemens	2.5 m/s	97.1%	100%
Shuang-Ming et al. [43]	2011	128	ARFI – Acuson S2000-Siemens	2.22 m/s	89.7%	95%
Zhang et al. [26]	2013	154	ARFI – Acuson S2000-Siemens	2.22 m/s	81.3%	93%
Park et al. [35]	2013	47	ARFI – Acuson S2000-Siemens	1.82 m/s	71.8%	75%
Kim et al. [36]*	2013	101	ARFI – Acuson S2000-Siemens	2.73 m/s	96.4%	65.8%
Guibal et al. [29]	2013	139	2D-SWE – Aixplorer-Supersonic Imagine	6 kPa	70,9%	30%
Zhang et al. [7]	2014	170	ARFI – Acuson S2000-Siemens	2.16 m/s	81.3%	71.4%
Guo et al. [67]	2015	134	ARFI – Acuson S2000-Siemens	2.13 m/s	83.3%	77.9%
Goya et al. [47]	2015	117	ARFI – Acuson S2000-Siemens	2.52 m/s	97%	66%
Lu et al. [57]	2015	373	ElastPQ – Philips-iU22	13 kPa	78%	83%
Park et al. [25]	2015	136	2D-SWE – Aixplorer-Supersonic Imagine	30.8 kPa	70.6%	82.4%
Tian et al. [24]	2016	229	2D-SWE – Aixplorer-Supersonic Imagine	39.6 kPa (Emax)	87.7%	83.7%
Dong et al. [34]	2017	154	ElastPQ – Philips-EPIQ7	2.06 m/s	80.6%	88%
Nagolu et al. [76]	2017	60	ARFI – Acuson S2000-Siemens	2 m/s	92%	96%
Gerber et al. [39]	2017	106	2D-SWE – Aixplorer-Supersonic Imagine	20.7 kPa	79%	62%
Grgurevic et al. [28]	2018	259	2D-SWE – Aixplorer-Supersonic Imagine	22.3 kPa	83%	86%
Akdoğan et al. [74]	2018	70	ARFI – Acuson S2000-Siemens	2.32 m/s	93%	60%

Study	Year	Number of lesions	Type of elastography –vendor	SWE value cut-off	Sensitivity	Specificity
Zhang et al. [42]	2020	104	ARFI – Acuson S2000-Siemens	1.95 m/s (Emax)	93%	92%
Serag et al. [50]*	2020	110	ElastPQ – Philips-iU22	13.24 kPa	78.0%	71.2%
Abdel-Latif et al. [59]	2020	75	2D-SWE – Logiq E9-GE healthcare	14.165 kPa	91.1%	78.3%
Singla et al. [46]	2020	50	ElastPQ – Philips-iU22	25 kPa	66%	30%
Youssef et al. [68]*	2022	138	2D-SWE – Logiq S8-XD Clear-GE Healthcare	11,13 kPa	100%	80%
Guo et al. [40]	2022	132	ElastPQ – Acuson Sequoia-Siemens	1.905 m/s (Emax)	71%	84.38%
Nacheva-Georgieva. [20]***	2022	125	2D-SWE, pSWE – Esoate MyLab 9 Exp	1.59 m/s	100%	100%

SWE value: Shear wave elasticity value. *Hemangiomas are compared to malignant FLLs only.*
Hemangiomas are compared to metastatic lesions only.
Hemangiomas compared to HCC only.

Table 3.
Sensitivity and specificity and shear wave elasticity cut-off values to discriminate benign from malignant FLLs from some of the studies that reported statistically significance in differentiation for ultrasound elastography.

Absolute stiffness values consistently achieve higher diagnostic accuracy compared to RR. For example, Guo et al. reported a SWV cut-off of 2.13 m/s and a RR of 1.37 m/s with an AUROC of 0.824 for SWV vs. an AUROC of 0.660 for RR. SWV outperformed RR measurements [67]. In the study by Dong et al. RR cut-off value to differentiate a malignant lesion from a benign was 1,67 with a sensitivity of 67,3% and specificity of 71,2%. But the sensitivity and specificity for RR were lower than absolute elasticity of FLLs, which were 80,6% and 88% respectively [34]. Similar observations were made by Tian et al. [24]. Grgurevic et al. reported that stiffness ratio of the FLL to the liver and stiffness variance both had a lesser AUROC of 0,58 and 0,62 compared to absolute SWV of FLL [28]. Lu et al. found a stiffness cut-off of 13 kPa (AUROC 0.86) was superior to RR of 1,3 (AUROC 0.69) for differentiating benign and malignant lesions [57]. In the metanalysis by Hu et al. which incorporated data from 15 studies, the pooled sensitivity and specificity of stiffness relative ratio using a cut-off value of 1.3–1.67 were 0.72% (95% CI: 0.59–0.83) and 0.82% (95% CI: 0.43–0.97), respectively, with a summary ROC of 0.78% (95% CI: 0.74–0.81) which were slightly lower than the values for absolute elastography measurements of FLLs [22].

Alternative approaches, such as summing or subtracting stiffness values between lesions and parenchyma, have shown promise. Park et al. demonstrated summed SWV values significantly enhanced diagnostic differentiation (AUROC 0.853) [35].

Study	SWE Benign FLL	Benign RR	SWE Malignant FLL	Malignant RR	Accuracy	AUROC
Cho et al. [62]*	1.51 ± 0.71 m/s		2.45 ± 0.81 m/s			
Davies et al. [43]**	1.35 ± 0.48 m/s		4.23 ± 0.59 m/s			0.999
Shuang-Ming et al. [29]	1.47 ± 0.53 m/s		3.16 ± 0.80 m/s.		92.2%	0.95 (95%CI:0.92–0.99)
Zhang et al. [26]	1.33 ± 0.38 m/s		2.59 ± 0.91 m/S			0.91 (95%CI:0.87–0.96)
Park et al. [35]	1.51 ± 0.69 m/s		2.31 ± 1.05 m/s			0.853 (95%CI:0.745–0.960)
Kim et al. [36]*	1.80 ± 0.57 m/s		2.66 ± 0.94 m/s			0.86
Zhang et al. [7]	1.78 ± 0.68 m/s		2.93 ± 0.87 m/s		78.8%	0.84 (95%CI:0.78–0.91)
Guo et al. [67]	1.69 ± 0.89 m/s	1.26 ± 0.78 m/s	2.95 ± 1.00 m/s	1.83 ± 1.33 m/s		0.824 (95%CI:0.748–0.899)
Goya et al. [47]	2.38 ± 1.08 m/s		3.36 ± 0.72 m/s)			0,797 (95%CI:0.708–0.886)
Lu et al. [57]	8.4 (2.9–49) kPa	1.6 (0.3–6.7)	21 (4.4–188) kPa	2.5 (0.5–37)		0.86 (95%CI:0.81–0.90)
Park et al. [25]	22.05 ± 17.24 kPa	7.14 ± 6.99 kPa	60.41 ± 41.81 kPa	3.7 ± 3.77 kPa		0.793
Tian et al. [24]*	25.75 ± 15.64 kPa		72.60 ± 38.94 kPa			0.920 (95%CI:0.872–0.953)
Dong et al. [34]	1.57 ± 0.55 m/s	2.23 ± 0.49	2.77 ± 0.68 m/s	2.23 ± 0.49 m/s		0.704
Nagolu et al. [76]	1.30 ± 0.35 m/s		2.93 ± 0.75 m/s,			0.877 (95%CI:0.777–0.976)
Gerber et al. [39]	16.4(2,1-71,9) kPa		36(4,1-142,9) kPa			0,73
Akdoğan et al. [74]	2.26 ± 0.78 m/s		3.31 ± 0.65 m/s			0.826
Zhang et al. [42]*	1.30 ± 0.46 m/s		3.29 ± 0.88 m/s		92.3%	0.978
Serag et al. [50]*	10.32 ± 6.74 kPa		17.23 ± 8.25 kPa		64.2%	0.777
Abdel-Latif et al. [59]	10.68 kPa		20.22 kPa		92%	0.834
Youssef et al. [68]	9.36 ± 2.48 kPa	1.86 ± 0.62	22.53 ± 9.33 kPa	2.53 ± 1.31	95.7%	0.989
Guo et al. [40]	2.21 ± 0.57 m/s		1.59 ± 0.37 m/s		74.24%	0.843
Nacheva-Georgieva et al. [20]***	0.78–1.62 m/s		2.52–4.43 m/s		100%	1.00

*Emax values are used instead of Emean. (−): not provided. Hemangiomas are compared to malignant FLLs only.
**Hemangiomas are compared to metastatic lesions only. ***Hemangiomas compared to HCC only.

Table 4.
Results from some of the studies that include shear wave elasticity (SWE) values of benign focal liver lesions (FLL) and malignant FLL including relative ratio (RR) of SWE values of benign FLL divided by SWE values of surrounding parenchyma and RR of SWE value of malignant FLL divided by SWE value of surrounding parenchyma and the accuracy of the study and area under the curve (AUROC) values.

Kim et al. suggested differences in SWV could better distinguish hepatocellular carcinoma (HCC) from other malignancies (**Table 4**) [36].

In cirrhotic livers, stiffness ratios may aid in evaluating HCC and ICC [24]. Guibal et al. using stiffness ratio predicted HCC with 65% sensitivity and 93% specificity [29]. Tian et al. advocated for comparing absolute liver stiffness values to standardized benchmarks to enhance diagnostic accuracy [24]. In the study by Lu et al., the stiffness ratio proved more effective than stiffness values in differentiating metastases from primary liver cancers (HCCs and ICCs), achieving an AUROC of 0.71 compared to 0.58. It also demonstrated greater accuracy in distinguishing cirrhotic nodules from other benign lesions, with an AUROC of 0.86 compared to 0.53 [57]. While ratios may improve differentiation in specific cases, absolute stiffness measurements remain the preferred parameter for elastographic studies of FLLs (**Table 5**) [28, 52, 57, 68].

9. Benign liver lesions

Cystic liver lesions are well-defined, avascular, and anechoic on B-mode ultrasound, with low stiffness values in elastography. For example, Abdel-Latif et al. reported stiffness values of 0 for simple cysts [59]. Complicated cysts, such as those with debris or infection, may mimic solid lesions. Park et al. found complicated cysts had an Emean of 3.9 ± 4.8 kPa, indicating softness compared to liver parenchyma [25]. Similarly, Gad et al. observed an elasticity of 1.48 kPa for inflammatory lesions [27]. Abscesses exhibit a wide stiffness range. Park et al. reported abscesses with an Emean of 22.13 ± 5.14 kPa and a relative ratio (RR) of 4.11 ± 3.83, indicating hard lesions [25]. Conversely, Shuang Ming et al. observed low SWV values (<2.22 m/s) in abscesses [43].

Study	Year	Type of elastography	Number of lesions B/M	Mean SWE value for benign FLL	Mean SWE value for malignant FLL
Heide et al. [33]	2010	ARFI – Acuson S2000-Siemens	62 (38/24)	2.60 ± 0.97 m/s	2.90 ± 1.16 m/s
Gallotti et al. [48]	2012	ARFI – Acuson S2000-Siemens	40 (25/25)	2,32 m/s	2,59 m/s
Frulio et al. [30]	2013	ARFI – Acuson S2000-Siemens	79 (43/36)	2.53 ± 0.83 m/s	2.60 ± 1.15 m/s
Guibal et al. [29]*	2013	2D-SWE – Aixplorer -Supersonic Imagine	139 (53/86)	18.53 ± 13.5 kPa	26.9 ± 18.8 kPa
Ronot et al. [45]	2015	2D-SWE – Aixplorer -Supersonic Imagine	105 (102/3)	26.7 ± 14 kPa	29.3 ± 9.7 kPa
Hasab-Allah. [52]	2017	ElastPQ – Philips-iU22	197 (18/179)	7.45 ± 4.56 kPa	10.71 ± 3.81 kPa
Singla et al. [46]*	2020	ElastPQ – Philips-iU22	50 (14/36)	3,28 kPa	4,83 kPa
Serag et al. [50]*	2020	ElastPQ – Philips-iU22	110 (28/82)	10.32 ± 6.74 kPa	17.23 ± 8.25 kPa
Gad et al. [27]	2021	ElastPQ – Philips-iU22	80 (25/54)	5.08 kPa	5.51 kPa

SWE: shear wave elasticity value, B/M: no. of benign FLL/no. of malignant FLL. *The difference between Emean of benign and malignant FLLs were statistically significant but with limited discriminatory effectiveness, low sensitivity, low specificity and accuracy.*

Table 5.
Some studies which concluded that elastography is statistically insignificant in distinguishing malignant from benign FLL.

Abdel-Latif et al. reported low Emean values of 8.79 kPa for hydatid cysts [59]. Goya et al. noted that late-stage hydatid cysts and Fasciola hepatica lesions showed high SWV values compared to early lesions, ranging from 3.35 to 4.83 m/s [47]. Focal fatty sparing (FFS) can resemble focal liver lesions (FLLs) but is softer than surrounding liver parenchyma. Heide et al. reported an SWV of 1.02 ± 1.16 m/s for FFS [33], while Park et al. found an Emean of 15.15 ± 11.38 kPa and an RR of 2.3 ± 0.77 for FFS [25]. Focal fatty infiltration (FFI) also demonstrates variable stiffness, with studies reporting Emean values ranging from 8.5 to 11.2 kPa [50, 59]. Hematomas and scars exhibit high stiffness values, with Park et al. reporting 31.05 ± 1.34 kPa for hematomas and Guibal et al. recording 52.7 ± 4.7 kPa for scars [25, 29].

9.1 Hepatic hemangiomas (HH)

Hepatic hemangiomas (HHs), the most common benign mesenchymal liver tumors, occur in 10–20% of the population [23]. Composed of endothelial cells, they appear as hyperechoic or isoechoic, well-circumscribed lesions on ultrasound but may present heterogeneously with growth or in cases of steatosis or sclerosis. US has a sensitivity of 96.9% and specificity of 60.3% for diagnosing HHs, but distinguishing them from metastatic lesions or HCCs can be challenging, particularly when they appear hypoechoic [69]. CDUS often fails to show vascularity due to the slow flow within HHs, while CEUS reveals characteristic arterial-phase enhancement with no washout in later phases [1, 69]. Elastography typically shows HHs as soft lesions with SWV values of 1.3–1.83 m/s, though some studies report higher values [33, 35, 67]. Variability in stiffness is attributed to structural changes like thrombosis, sclerosis, or calcification [33, 35, 47]. Studies using 2D-SWE report Emean values ranging from 4.9 to 14.1 kPa for HHs, with higher values noted in cases with histological alterations [28, 52, 56]. Relative elasticity ratios (RR) for HHs are generally slightly above or comparable to surrounding liver tissue [23, 36, 67]. Using SWV cut-offs improves differentiation between HHs and malignant lesions. Davies et al. reported an SWV cut-off of 1.0 m/s, achieving 97.1% sensitivity and 100% specificity [23]. Similarly, Cho et al. found a 2 m/s cut-off provided 74% sensitivity and 81% specificity for distinguishing

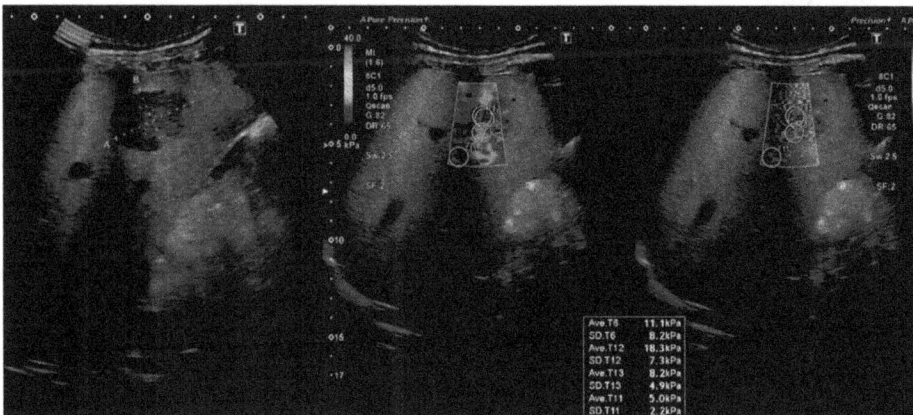

Figure 1.
An atypical hemangioma lesion in a 43-year-old male patient appearing hypoechoic on B-mode ultrasound displaying a low Emean stiffness value of 12.5 kPa compared to the normal appearing liver background with SWE of 5.0 kPa.

HHs from malignant lesions [44]. Park et al. reported an Emean of 12.91 ± 9.42 kPa and an RR of 2.86 ± 2.07 for HHs, supporting SWE's diagnostic utility [25].

Studies on pediatric HHs show higher Emean values. Wang et al. reported 19.0 ± 16 kPa for HHs versus 58.4 ± 19.5 kPa for hepatoblastomas, with a 2D-SWE cut-off of 39.5 kPa achieving 88.1% sensitivity and 86.2% specificity [51, 70]. Ozmen et al. similarly reported a cut-off of 23.62 kPa to differentiate HHs from hepatoblastomas and HCCs (**Figure 1**) [71].

9.2 Focal nodular hyperplasia (FNH)

FNH is the second most common benign liver lesion, accounting for 25% of benign FLLs. It typically appears as a well-circumscribed, iso- or hypoechoic lesion with a hyperechoic central scar. On CDUS, a spoke-wheel vascular pattern is often observed [72, 73]. FNH predominantly occurs in young women and may coexist with HHs (23%) or HAs (3.6%) [72]. On CEUS, FNH displays centrifugal arterial filling with persistent portal and venous enhancement, achieving sensitivity and specificity of 80–100% and 85–95%, respectively [72, 73]. FNH typically exhibits the highest stiffness values among benign FLLs due to fibrotic composition, with Emean values reported as 33.3 ± 12.7 kPa by Ronot et al. [45] and 47 ± 31 kPa by Brunel et al. [73], and SWV values ranging from 2.75 to 3.22 m/s [45, 73, 74]. These values are significantly higher than HHs or inflammatory lesions [30, 73, 74]. Factors such as lesion size (<3 cm) and depth (>8 cm) can reduce measurement accuracy [73, 75].

Differentiation of FNH from HAs, which carry hemorrhage and malignancy risks, is critical [72]. Guibal et al. reported stiffness values and relative ratios (RR) as effective markers, with a cut-off of 9.7 kPa achieving 90% sensitivity and 93.7% specificity [29]. Brunel et al. demonstrated 95% diagnostic accuracy using an SWE stiffness cut-off of 18.8 kPa [73]. However, overlapping stiffness values between FNH and HAs, especially in smaller lesions, remain a challenge [30, 75]. Fibrolamellar HCCs can mimic FNH but typically show calcifications, invasion, lymphadenopathy, and higher stiffness values. On imaging, fibrolamellar HCCs exhibit rapid arterial enhancement and venous washout, with hypointense scars on T2-weighted MRI distinguishing them from hyperintense scars in FNH [72]. Stiffness values are significantly higher, with studies reporting SWVs up to 2.76 ± 1.75 m/s [47, 76]. While SWE enhances diagnostic accuracy, limitations such as interobserver variability and stiffness overlap necessitate combining it with modalities like CEUS and MRI, particularly for atypical cases [45, 73, 75].

9.3 Hepatocellular adenoma (HA)

HAs are rare benign liver lesions, most common in young women, with a prevalence of 0.05%. They are linked to estrogen exposure, oral contraceptives, and androgen use. Key risk factors for malignancy include male sex, lesion size >5 cm, and β-catenin activation. Up to 7% of HAs may progress to HCC, especially large lesions, but multiple HAs do not increase malignancy risk. Pregnancy increases bleeding risks, while lesion regression can occur with hormone cessation or menopause [75, 77]. HAs are molecularly classified into subtypes: inflammatory (iHAs), hepatocyte nuclear factor 1A- mutated (HNF1α-mutated), β-catenin-activated, and Sonic Hedgehog. iHAs (35% of cases) are linked to obesity and vascular congestion, while HNF1α-mutated HAs (35%) are associated with steatosis and lower malignant potential. β-Catenin-activated HAs (15–20%) have the highest risk of malignancy (up to 50%) and are often linked to anabolic steroid use [77].

On imaging, HAs show fast arterial fill-in with slow washout on CEUS and lack Kupffer cells, resulting in low hepatobiliary contrast on MRI. Sensitivity and specificity for MRI diagnosis range from 88 to 100%, but biopsy remains crucial for subtype differentiation [77]. HAs generally exhibit lower stiffness values on SWE compared to FNH [45, 73, 75]. Guibal et al. reported Emean values of 9.4 ± 4.3 kPa, while Ronot et al. noted 19.7 ± 9.8 kPa [29, 45]. These values reflect their pathological similarity to hepatocytes and lack of biliary ducts or portal spaces [29, 45, 48]. SWE achieves high accuracy in distinguishing HAs from FNH, with a stiffness cut-off of 18.8 kPa yielding 95% diagnostic accuracy [73]. Subtype differentiation using SWE is possible, as iHAs show higher stiffness than HNF1α-mutated HAs due to inflammation and vascular congestion [30, 45]. Ronot et al. found mean stiffness values of 24 ± 8 kPa for iHAs and 11.8 ± 7.7 kPa for HNF1α-mutated HAs, with AUROCs of 0.88 and 0.95, respectively [45]. However, other studies, such as Taimr et al., reported significant overlaps in stiffness values, particularly in smaller or regressed lesions, cautioning against sole reliance on SWE for diagnosis [75].

9.4 Cirrhotic (regenerative and dysplastic) nodules

Cirrhotic nodules (regenerative nodules (RNs) and dysplastic nodules (DNs)) often exhibit increased stiffness values overlapping with HCCs leading to diagnostic challenges [7, 33, 43, 57, 74, 78]. Zhang et al. reported SWV values of 2.48 ± 0.64 m/s for RNs [7]. According to the study by Lu et al., a stiffness ratio of 0.7 effectively differentiated cirrhotic nodules from benign lesions with an AUROC 0.86, surpassing the performance of absolute stiffness values of 8 kPa with an AUROC of 0.53 [57]. Li et al. showed that stiffness cut-off (9.8 kPa), stiffness difference (<1 kPa), and ratio (1.2) distinguished small HCCs from cirrhotic nodules with sensitivities of 62, 96, and 82% and specificities of 83, 50 and 90% respectively. Adding alpha-fetoprotein (AFP) improved diagnostic sensitivity to 100% with a balanced specificity [78]. Gheorghe et al. identified blue color intensity on sonoelastography maps (cut-off 128.9; AUROC 0.94) and hypervascularity on Doppler ultrasound as key predictors of HCC compared to cirrhotic nodules [54].

10. Malignant lesions of the liver

10.1 Hepatocellular carcinoma (HCC)

SWE is widely used for assessing fibrosis, portal hypertension, and steatosis in chronic liver disease, providing insights into HCC risk. Patients with liver stiffness >10 kPa have a fourfold higher risk of HCC, emphasizing the importance of surveillance [37, 79]. On CEUS, HCCs typically show arterial hyperenhancement and late-onset washout, but well-differentiated HCCs may deviate from this pattern, complicating diagnosis, especially for smaller nodules [37].

Most HCCs exhibit higher absolute and relative stiffness compared to benign lesions, with ARFI values ranging from 2.1 to 3.4 m/s, ElastPQ from 4.9 to 25.4 kPa, and 2D-SWE from 14.8 to 61.8 kPa [24, 25, 29, 60]. However, some HCCs may appear soft, with stiffness values overlapping with benign lesions such as RNs or HHs [7, 30, 48]. In cases of cirrhosis, HCCs may exhibit stiffness similar to the fibrotic liver, complicating differentiation [47, 57]. Studies by Akdoğan et al. and Gallotti et al. noted that some HCCs had relative ratios (RR) <1, reflecting heterogeneity and fibrosis variability in surrounding parenchyma [48, 74]. Relative stiffness ratios can aid in differentiating HCCs from metastatic cancers but are less reliable for distinguishing HCCs from benign lesions. Ghiuchici et al. observed that all 88 HCCs in their study were softer than the surrounding parenchyma, with a shear wave velocity (SWV) value of 2.16 ± 0.75 m/s and a relative ratio (RR) of 1.33 ± 0.66. The addition of SWE findings enhanced the diagnostic accuracy of CEUS, particularly in the 23.9% of HCC lesions that did not display a typical enhancement pattern [37]. Using RR of <1, Guibal et al. reported sensitivity, the specificity, the negative predictive value and the positive predictive value of 65, 93, 92 and 68% respectively for the diagnosis of HCC [29]. Dong et al. reported that RR cut-off value of 1.67 and an elasticity value of 2.06 m/s was significant in differentiating HCC from benign lesions [34]. But in the study by Park et al., RR of 3.76 did not help to differentiate HCC from benign lesions while absolute stiffness values did [25]. Tian et al. [24] and Guo et al. [67] reported similar observations [24, 67]. In the study by Lu et al., HCC lesions exhibited higher stiffness compared to benign lesions. Absolute stiffness values outperformed the relative stiffness ratio for distinguishing HCC from benign lesions, achieving an AUROC of 0.86 compared to 0.69. However, the stiffness ratios were valuable in differentiating HCC from metastatic cancers, with an AUROC of 0.71. Neither stiffness values nor stiffness ratios were effective in differentiating CCC from HCC. Authors observed significant peritumoral stiffness variation around the lesion, exceeding the intratumoral stiffness variability. Measurements taken 2 cm away from the lesion demonstrated less variability and were more reliable for diagnostic purposes [57].

HCCs may arise in non-cirrhotic livers due to nonalcoholic fatty liver disease (NAFLD), metabolic syndrome, viral infections or hereditary conditions. These HCCs often exhibit lower stiffness due to reduced fibrosis and ECM changes. Steatohepatitic and clear cell HCCs, for example, show softer stiffness due to high lipid or glycogen content. Conversely, aggressive subtypes like scirrhous or fibrolamellar HCCs exhibit higher stiffness due to fibrosis or mesenchymal changes [80]. Treatments such as sorafenib or transcatheter arterial chemoembolization (TACE) or transcatheter radioembolization (TARE) can alter tumor stiffness. Cell death and ischemia may reduce stiffness in tumor cores, while fibrosis and calcifications increase stiffness in peripheral regions [81]. Ablative therapies can stiffen tumors, but residual softer regions may indicate viable tumor areas [82–88]. Goya et al. reported

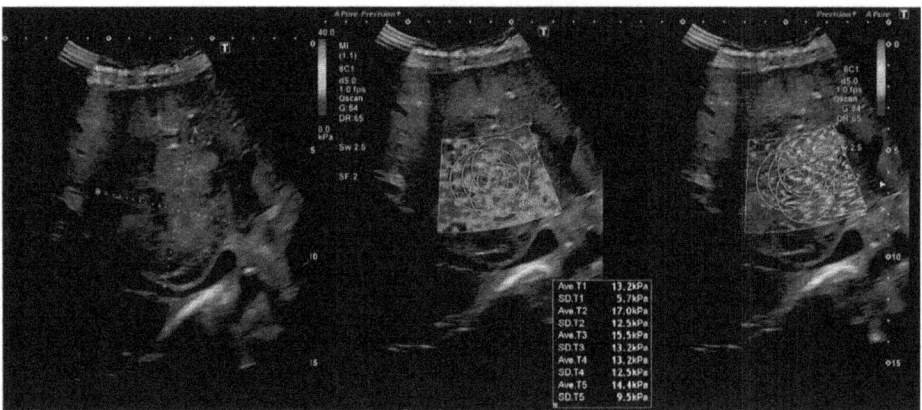

Figure 2.
Multifocal hepatocellular carcinoma in a 74-year-old female with relatively low stiffness values (Emean:14.6 kPa) in a relatively normal background liver tissue.

post- radiofrequency ablation (RFA) HCCs with high stiffness values [47]. HCCs are generally softer than metastatic lesions or cholangiocarcinomas (CCCs), though exceptions exist due to pathological variability. Studies by Hasab-Allah et al. and Lu et al. showed that relative stiffness ratios outperformed absolute values in distinguishing HCCs from metastases [52, 57], while others reported overlapping stiffness values across malignant lesions (**Figure 2**) [38, 47].

10.2 Intrahepatic cholangiocarcinoma (ICC)

ICC is the second most common primary liver tumor, accounting for 15–20% of cases [89]. While cirrhosis and hepatitis B/C infections are shared risk factors with HCC, cirrhosis is more strongly linked to HCC [67]. Elastography combined with CEUS can help differentiate ICC from HCC, though biopsy is often required for confirmation [49]. ICC is typically stiffer than HCC, with reported ARFI values ranging from 1.65 to 3.9 m/s [25, 26], ElastPQ values approximately 6.8–32 kPa [27, 50], and 2D-SWE values up to 96.2 kPa [24]. The increased stiffness is attributed to fibrotic tissue within ICC [25, 89]. However, ICCs in cirrhotic livers may present with lower stiffness than the surrounding parenchyma, as noted by Gad et al., who reported an Emean of 6.4 kPa and an RR of 0.56 for four ICCs [27].

Most studies report that ICC exhibits higher stiffness than HCC, with cut-offs aiding differentiation. Gerber et al. achieved 81% sensitivity and 71% specificity using a cut-off of 61.3 kPa [38], while Guibal et al. reported 92.3% sensitivity and 85.7% specificity at 27.5 kPa [29]. However, overlap in stiffness values between ICC and HCC has been observed in some studies [25, 47]. Ainora et al. used a multiparametric ultrasound (MP-US) approach, incorporating CEUS and SWE, to differentiate ICC from HCC. ICCs demonstrated higher stiffness (47.1 ± 14.4 kPa vs. 35.7 ± 13.8 kPa). Their predictive model achieved 92% sensitivity and 93% specificity [49]. A meta-analysis by Mohebbi et al. that included 18 studies and 1057 patients revealed Emean values of 28,3 kPa for 863 HCC lesions and 44.0 kPa for 188 ICC lesions. ICC lesions were 34.3% stiffer than HCCs, while surrounding parenchyma was 75% stiffer in HCC. The combined sensitivity and specificity for differentiation were 87 and 82%, with an AUROC of 0.90 [89]. Conversely, Lu et al. found no clear distinction between

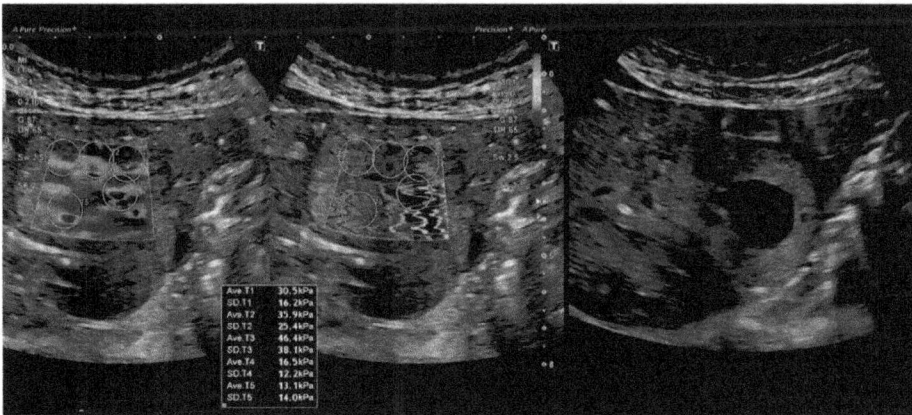

Figure 3.
A cholangiocarcinoma lesion in a cirrhotic female patient exhibiting variant heterogenecity and central cystic necrotic changes. Emean is 28.5 kPa.

HCC and ICC using SWE due to overlapping stiffness values, though SWE effectively differentiated malignant from benign lesions (**Figure 3**) [57].

10.3 Metastatic lesions

Metastatic lesions exhibit high stiffness values which can sometimes overlap with CCC. Gallotti et al. [48] reported a mean SWV of 2.87 ± 1.13 m/s [51], while Frulio et al. [30] and Akdoğan et al. observed higher values of 3.0 ± 1.35 m/s and 3.59 ± 0.51 m/s, with breast cancer metastases being the stiffest [30, 48, 74]. Although metastatic lesions generally have higher stiffness than HCC, Choong et al. found no significant difference, with mean Emean values of 51.45 kPa for HCC and 49.89 kPa for metastases. A cut-off of 18.25 kPa effectively differentiated malignant FLLs from normal liver tissue [38]. Abdel-Latif et al. noted colon cancer metastases were softer than breast cancer [59], and

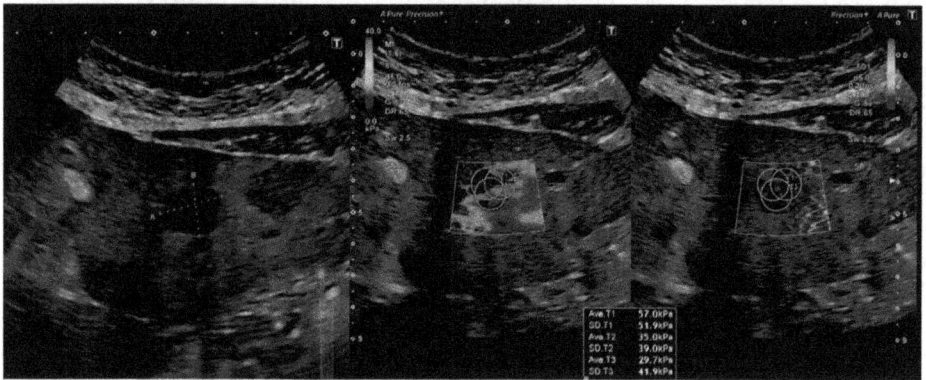

Figure 4.
Hypoechoic metastasis from invasive ductal carcinoma of the breast in the left lobe of the liver displaying very high stiffness values (Emean: 40.7 kPa).

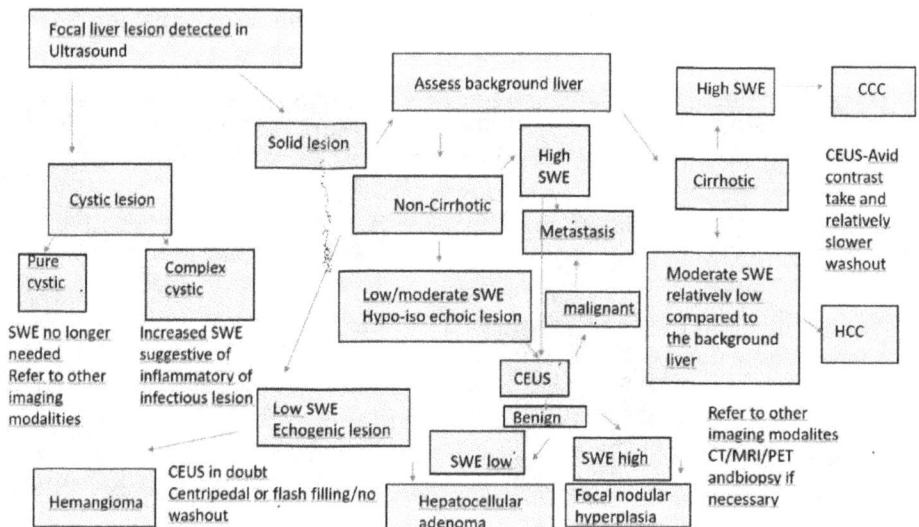

Figure 5.
Diagnostic flowchart for ultrasound elastography of focal liver lesions.

Guibal et al. reported neuroendocrine metastases were stiffer than adenocarcinomas [29]. Relative stiffness ratio (RR) has been more effective than absolute stiffness in distinguishing metastases from primary liver tumors. Lu et al. achieved an AUROC of 0.71 using RR [49], while Dong et al. found an RR cut-off of 1.67 offered greater accuracy than absolute stiffness values in differentiation of HCC from metastatic lesions [56]. These findings highlight the diagnostic value of RR in this context (**Figures 4** and **5**).

11. Utilization in ablative therapies

Successful tumor ablation requires complete tumor coverage in a single session, as incomplete ablation increases recurrence risk [6, 83]. CEUS is commonly used intra-procedurally to detect residual tumors, identified by contrast uptake. However, CEUS's availability, cost, and software requirements can limit its use. Contrast-enhanced CT and MRI, typically performed a month later due to delayed perilesional hyperemia resolution, can delay further treatment [6, 83]. SWE, especially 3D-SWE, has emerged as a real-time alternative for assessing ablation. By measuring tissue stiffness changes post-ablation, SWE identifies ablated zones, with stiffness highest centrally (59.1 kPa), decreasing toward transitional (13.1 kPa) and normal tissue zones (4.3 kPa). A cut-off of 13.1 kPa differentiates viable from ablated tissue [21]. Bo et al. showed SWE effectively visualizes ablation zones, correlating with ablation specimens. These stiffness changes persist, enabling immediate treatment evaluation without waiting weeks for hyperemia resolution [83–85].

Liver stiffness assessment can predict prognosis and HCC recurrence. Stiffness values >13 kPa are linked to poor outcomes. Lee et al. found 2D-SWE stiffness >13.3 kPa associated with poorer survival in 134 patients undergoing RFA [86]. Yoon et al. identified ARFI and TE cut-offs (1.6 m/s and 14.0 kPa) linked to higher recurrence risks, with sensitivities and specificities of 65.2–84.3% [87]. Liver stiffness >11.75 kPa increases liver failure risk post-resection, favoring alternative therapies like TARE or TACE for high-risk patients [90]. Praktiknjo et al. observed that baseline stiffness >17.5 kPa in responding HCC lesions predicted higher non-target recurrence risk (sensitivity 100% and specificity 83.3%). Elevated HCC stiffness may indicate aggressive behavior and neoangiogenesis, although liver stiffness showed no such correlation [88].

12. Guidance and assistance to biopsy of focal lesions

Stiffness values, which reflect the pathological composition of tissues, can guide biopsies to the most active and viable areas of a lesion, avoiding cystic or necrotic regions and thereby improving the diagnostic accuracy of the biopsy sample. In cases of focal liver lesions (FLLs) with ambiguous stiffness values near the malignancy cut-off, a biopsy may be warranted for definitive diagnosis. Additionally, persistent stiffness in a malignant lesion following ablative, systemic, or intra-arterial therapies may indicate the need for a biopsy to assess recurrence or inadequate treatment response [82, 88].

13. Role of AI in SWE of FLLs

AI has the capability to analyze and interpret vast amounts of data, offering the potential to refine cut-off values and suggest specific diagnoses. Advanced techniques such as radiomics, segmentation, and machine learning can detect subtle changes that are imperceptible to the human eye. Automated reports can be generated from complex calculations, and stiffness data can be seamlessly integrated with other diagnostic studies for more precise results. By reducing user-related biases, artifacts, and interobserver variability, AI enhances the reliability of elastography. Acting as a "virtual touch biopsy," AI can estimate the likelihood of malignancy, monitor stiffness trends over time to provide prognostic insights, and assess therapy response, flagging lesions that are unresponsive to treatment for further evaluation [4]. An example is in the study by Wang et al. who used radiomics analysis in SWE evaluation of 175 FLLs and improvement in diagnostic accuracy is noted compared to conventional stiffness analysis with an AUROC of 0.94 to 0.92 respectively [5]. Another example is the study by Shen et al., which evaluated 262 patients using a non-invasive predictive nomogram based on training and test set data derived from the combination of Sonazoid CEUS and Sound Touch Elastography (STE). The nomogram incorporated variables such as ALT levels, arterial phase hyperenhancement (APHE), Kupffer phase enhancement, and lesion stiffness. The nomogram demonstrated excellent performance, achieving an AUROC of 0.988, with sensitivity and specificity of 94.6 and 95.2%, respectively, in the test set [91].

14. Emerging technologies

Tissue scatterer distribution imaging (TSI) is an innovative ultrasound technology that mathematically analyzes the distribution of backscattered signals, focusing on tissue microstructure and heterogeneity. Unlike conventional methods, TSI is highly reliable for image capture and is unaffected by factors such as lesion size, depth, or motion artifacts, as it primarily depends on image quality and signal-to-noise ratio. In a study by Chen et al., on differentiation of 61 benign and 204 malignant FLLs, median TSI values were significantly lower for malignant lesions (0.62) compared to TSI of benign lesions (0.74) and with a cut-off value of 0.67, TSI achieved an AUROC of 0.78–0.83 compared to 0.84 for SWE highlighting its potential as a complementary technology [92].

Shear Wave Dispersion Imaging (SWDI) measures tissue viscoelastic properties by analyzing the attenuation of propagating shear waves. Unlike SWE, which focuses on stiffness, SWDI assesses viscosity, tissue fluidity, inflammation, necrosis, and cellular composition. SWDI is expressed as frequency-dependent dispersion (m/s/kHz). SWDI and SWE are complementary studies, offering unique insights into malignancy potential and prognostic behavior of FLLs. Dong et al. studied 58 patients using the Canon Aplio i900 ultrasound system and reported significantly higher viscosity values in malignant lesions (14.79 ± 3.15 m/s/kHz) compared to benign lesions (13.36 ± 2.76 m/s/kHz). With a viscosity cut-off of 13.15 m/s/kHz, SWDI achieved a sensitivity of 83.3% and specificity of 56.5%, with an AUROC of 0.71. Among malignant lesions, metastatic tumors had the highest viscosity values [93].

SWDI is less effective than SWE for diagnosing severe fibrosis and cirrhosis, showing stronger correlations with necroinflammatory changes rather than steatosis. For liver fibrosis staging, a cut-off value of 12.7 m/s/kHz was identified in a study involving 210 HCC patients who underwent liver resection [94]. Schulz et al. compared 2D-SWE, SWDI, and Attenuation Imaging (ATI) in 22 patients with primary biliary cholangitis (PBC) in a pioneering study, and they found that 2D-SWE significantly correlated with fibrosis markers such as platelet count, spleen length, and fibrosis scores, while SWDI correlated with alkaline phosphatase, a key prognostic marker in PBC, with a median value of 13.9 m/s/kHz. ATI, however, which quantifies liver steatosis, showed no significant correlation [95].

15. Conclusions

In conclusion; SWE is a helpful diagnostic and prognostic tool in the evaluation and management of liver lesions, particularly in differentiation of FNH from HA and in differentiation of malignant lesions such as HCC and CCC. Its ability to quantitatively assess tissue stiffness provides critical insights into disease severity, risk of malignancy, and treatment response. While SWE's diagnostic accuracy is enhanced when combined with other modalities like CEUS. The variability in stiffness values, influenced by tumor composition, surrounding tissue, and therapeutic interventions, highlights the complexity of liver pathology and the importance of integrating multiple diagnostic parameters. SWE's role in liver imaging continues to evolve, with future implementation of AI imaging, SWE will be offering valuable real-time guidance in personalized patient management and treatment planning.

Conflict of interest

The authors declare no conflict of interest.

Appendices and nomenclature

FLLs	Focal liver lesions
CT	Computed tomography
MRI	Magnetic resonance imaging
PET-CT	Positron emission tomography computed tomography
US	Ultrasound
CEUS	Contrast-enhanced ultrasound
SWE	Shear wave elastography
ECM	Extracellular matrix
EFSUMB	European Federation of Societies for Ultrasound in Medicine and Biology
WFUMB	World Federation for Ultrasound in Medicine and Biology
SE	Strain elastography
ETLT	Elasticity type of liver tumor
TE	Transient elastography
ARFI	Acoustic radiation force impulse
1D-SWE	One dimensional shear save elastography
VTI	Virtual touch imaging
p-SWE	Point SWE
ROI	Region of interest
2D-SWE	Two dimensional SWE
m/s	Meter per second
kPa	KiloPascals
3D-SWE	Three dimensional SWE
VTQ	Virtual touch quantification

SRU	Society of radiologists in ultrasound
SWV	Shear wave velocity
IQR	Interquartile range
SD	Standard deviation
Emean	Mean elasticity
Emin	Minimum elasticity
Emax	Maximum elasticity
PACS	Picture archiving and communication system
HHs	Hemangiomas
FNHs	Focal nodular hyperplasias
CNs	Cirrhotic nodules
HAs	Hepatocellular adenomas
CCCs	Cholangiocarcinomas
HCCs	Hepatocellular carcinomas
CDUS	Color Doppler Ultrasound
PD-1	Programmed cell death protein 1
AUROC	Area under the curve
E-SD	Elasticity SD
RR	Relative elasticity ratio
FFS	Focal fatty sparing
FFI	Focal fatty infiltration
iHAs	Inflammatory Hepatic Adenomas
HNF1α-mutated	Hepatocyte nuclear factor 1A- mutated
RNs	Regenerative nodules
DNs	Dysplastic nodules
AFP	alpha-fetoprotein
NAFLD	Nonalcoholic fatty liver disease
TACE	Transcatheter arterial chemoembolization
TARE	Transcatheter radioembolization
RFA	Radiofrequency ablation
ICC	Intrahepatic cholangiocarcinoma
MP-US	Multiparametric ultrasound
STE	Sound touch elastography
APHE	Arterial phase hyperenhancement
TSI	Tissue scatterer distribution imaging
SWDI	Shear wave dispersion imaging

Author details

Evren Üstüner*, Kemal Altınbaş and Metin Yavuz
Department of Radiology, Ankara University Faculty of Medicine, Ultrasound Unit,
Ankara, Turkiye

*Address all correspondence to: evrenustuner@gmail.com

IntechOpen

References

[1] Bartolotta TV, Taibbi A, Randazzo A, Gagliardo C. New frontiers in liver ultrasound: From mono to multi parametricity. World Journal of Gastrointestinal Oncology. 2021;**13**(10):1302-1316. DOI: 10.4251/wjgo.v13.i10.1302

[2] Leow KS, Kwok CY, Low HM, Lohan R, Lim TC, Low SCA, et al. Algorithm-based approach to focal liver lesions in contrast-enhanced ultrasound. Australasian Journal of Ultrasound in Medicine. 2022;**25**(3):142-153. DOI: 10.1002/ajum.12306

[3] Jung EM, Dong Y, Jung F. Current aspects of multimodal ultrasound liver diagnostics using contrast-enhanced ultrasonography (CEUS), fat evaluation, fibrosis assessment, and perfusion analysis - An update. Clinical Hemorheology and Microcirculation. 2023;**83**(2):181-193. DOI: 10.3233/CH-239100

[4] Berzigotti A, Ferraioli G, Bota S, Gilja OH, Dietrich CF. Novel ultrasound-based methods to assess liver disease: The game has just begun. Digestive and Liver Disease. 2018;**50**(2):107-112. DOI: 10.1016/j.dld.2017.11.019

[5] Wang W, Zhang JC, Tian WS, Chen LD, Zheng Q, Hu HT, et al. Shear wave elastography-based ultrasomics: Differentiating malignant from benign focal liver lesions. Abdominal Radiology (NY). 2021;**46**(1):237-248. DOI: 10.1007/s00261-020-02614-3

[6] Conti CB, Cavalcoli F, Fraquelli M, Conte D, Massironi S. Ultrasound elastographic techniques in focal liver lesions. World Journal of Gastroenterology. 2016;**22**(9):2647-2656. DOI: 10.3748/wjg.v22.i9.2647

[7] Zhang P, Zhou P, Tian SM, Qian Y, Li JL, Li RZ. Diagnostic performance of contrast-enhanced sonography and acoustic radiation force impulse imaging in solid liver lesions. Journal of Ultrasound in Medicine. 2014;**33**(2):205-214. DOI: 10.7863/ultra.33.2.205

[8] Deng B, Zhao Z, Kong W, Han C, Shen X, Zhou C. Biological role of matrix stiffness in tumor growth and treatment. Journal of Translational Medicine. 2022;**20**(1):540. DOI: 10.1186/s12967-022-03768-y

[9] Gargalionis AN, Papavassiliou KA, Papavassiliou AG. Mechanobiology of solid tumors. Biochimica et Biophysica Acta - Molecular Basis of Disease. 2022;**1868**(12):166555. DOI: 10.1016/j.bbadis.2022.166555

[10] Barr RG. Shear wave liver elastography. Abdominal Radiology (NY). 2018;**43**(4):800-807. DOI: 10.1007/s00261-017-1375-1

[11] Dietrich CF, Bamber J, Berzigotti A, Bota S, Cantisani V, Castera L, et al. EFSUMB guidelines and recommendations on the clinical use of liver ultrasound elastography, update 2017 (long version). Ultraschall in der Medizin. 2017;**38**(4):e16-e47. DOI: 10.1055/s-0043-103952. Erratum in: Ultraschall Med. 2017 Aug;38(4):e48, 10.1055/a-0641-0076

[12] Ferraioli G, Barr RG, Berzigotti A, Sporea I, Wong VW, Reiberger T, et al. WFUMB guideline/guidance on liver multiparametric ultrasound: Part 1. Update to 2018 guidelines on liver ultrasound elastography. Ultrasound in Medicine & Biology. 2024;**50**(8):1071-1087. DOI: 10.1016/j.ultrasmedbio.2024.03.013

[13] Ferraioli G, Wong VW, Castera L, Berzigotti A, Sporea I, Dietrich CF, et al. Liver ultrasound elastography: An update to the world federation for ultrasound in medicine and biology guidelines and recommendations. Ultrasound in Medicine & Biology. 2018;**44**(12):2419-2440. DOI: 10.1016/j.ultrasmedbio.2018.07.008

[14] Piscaglia F, Marinelli S, Bota S, Serra C, Venerandi L, Leoni S, et al. The role of ultrasound elastographic techniques in chronic liver disease: Current status and future perspectives. European Journal of Radiology. 2014;**83**(3):450-455. DOI: 10.1016/j.ejrad.2013.06.009

[15] Sigrist RMS, Liau J, Kaffas AE, Chammas MC, Willmann JK. Ultrasound elastography: Review of techniques and clinical applications. Theranostics. 2017;**7**(5):1303-1329. DOI: 10.7150/thno.18650

[16] Kato K, Sugimoto H, Kanazumi N, Nomoto S, Takeda S, Nakao A. Intra-operative application of real-time tissue elastography for the diagnosis of liver tumours. Liver International. 2008;**28**(9):1264-1271. DOI: 10.1111/j.1478-3231.2008.01701.x

[17] Omichi K, Inoue Y, Hasegawa K, Sakamoto Y, Okinaga H, Aoki T, et al. Differential diagnosis of liver tumours using intraoperative real-time tissue elastography. The British Journal of Surgery. 2015;**102**(3):246-253. DOI: 10.1002/bjs.9728

[18] Sporea I, Bota S, Grădinaru-Tașcău O, Şirli R, Popescu A. Comparative study between two point shear wave elastographic techniques: Acoustic radiation force impulse (ARFI) elastography and ElastPQ. Medical Ultrasonography. 2014;**16**(4):309-314. DOI: 10.11152/mu.201.3.2066.164.isp1

[19] Naganuma H, Ishida H, Uno A, Nagai H, Kuroda H, Ogawa M. Diagnostic problems in two-dimensional shear wave elastography of the liver. World Journal of Radiology. 2020;**12**(5):76-86. DOI: 10.4329/wjr.v12.i5.76

[20] Nacheva-Georgieva EL, Doykov DI, Andonov VN, Doykova KA, Tsvetkova SB. Point shear wave elastography and 2-dimensional shear wave elastography as a non-invasive method in differentiating benign from malignant lesions. Gastroenterology Insights. 2022;**13**:129-304. DOI: 10.3390/gastroent13030030

[21] Sugimoto K, Oshiro H, Ogawa S, Honjo M, Hara T, Moriyasu F. Radiologic-pathologic correlation of three-dimensional shear-wave elastographic findings in assessing the liver ablation volume after radiofrequency ablation. World Journal of Gastroenterology. 2014;**20**(33):11850-11855. DOI: 10.3748/wjg.v20.i33.11850

[22] Hu X, Huang X, Chen H, Zhang T, Hou J, Song A, et al. Diagnostic effect of shear wave elastography imaging for differentiation of malignant liver lesions: A meta-analysis. BMC Gastroenterology. 2019;**19**(1):60. DOI: 10.1186/s12876-019-0976-2

[23] Davies G, Koenen M. Acoustic radiation force impulse elastography in distinguishing hepatic haemangiomata from metastases: Preliminary observations. The British Journal of Radiology. 2011;**84**(1006):939-943. DOI: 10.1259/bjr/97637841

[24] Tian WS, Lin MX, Zhou LY, Pan FS, Huang GL, Wang W, et al. Maximum value measured by 2-D shear wave elastography helps in differentiating malignancy from benign focal liver lesions. Ultrasound in Medicine

& Biology. 2016;**42**(9):2156-2166. DOI: 10.1016/j.ultrasmedbio.2016.05.002

[25] Park HS, Kim YJ, Yu MH, Jung SI, Jeon HJ. Shear wave elastography of focal liver lesion: Intraobserver reproducibility and elasticity characterization. Ultrasound Quarterly. 2015;**31**(4):262-271. DOI: 10.1097/ RUQ.0000000000000175

[26] Zhang P, Zhou P, Tian SM, Qian Y, Deng J, Zhang L. Application of acoustic radiation force impulse imaging for the evaluation of focal liver lesion elasticity. Hepatobiliary & Pancreatic Diseases International. 2013;**12**(2):165-170. DOI: 10.1016/s1499-3872(13)60027-2

[27] Gad MAM, Eraky TE, Omar HM, Abosheaishaa HM. Role of real-time shear-wave elastography in differentiating hepatocellular carcinoma from other hepatic focal lesions. European Journal of Gastroenterology & Hepatology. 2021;**33**(3):407-414. DOI: 10.1097/MEG.0000000000001741

[28] Grgurevic I, Bokun T, Salkic NN, Brkljacic B, Vukelić-Markovic M, Stoos-Veic T, et al. Liver elastography malignancy prediction score for noninvasive characterization of focal liver lesions. Liver International. 2018;**38**(6):1055-1063. DOI: 10.1111/ liv.13611

[29] Guibal A, Boularan C, Bruce M, Vallin M, Pilleul F, Walter T, et al. Evaluation of shear wave elastography for the characterisation of focal liver lesions on ultrasound. European Radiology. 2013;**23**(4):1138-1149. DOI: 10.1007/ s00330-012-2692-y

[30] Frulio N, Laumonier H, Carteret T, Laurent C, Maire F, Balabaud C, et al. Evaluation of liver tumors using acoustic radiation force impulse elastography and correlation with histologic data.

Journal of Ultrasound in Medicine. 2013;**32**(1):121-130. DOI: 10.7863/ jum.2013.32.1.121

[31] Tian S, Li H, Li R, Ran L, Li S, Wu J, et al. Prevalence of hepatic steatosis and metabolic associated fatty liver disease among female breast cancer survivors. Chinese Medical Journal. 2022;**135**(19):2372-2374. DOI: 10.1097/ CM9.0000000000002121

[32] Hwang JA, Jeong WK, Song KD, Kang KA, Lim HK. 2-D shear wave elastography for focal lesions in liver phantoms: Effects of background stiffness, depth and size of focal lesions on stiffness measurement. Ultrasound in Medicine & Biology. 2019;**45**(12):3261-3268. DOI: 10.1016/j. ultrasmedbio.2019.08.006

[33] Heide R, Strobel D, Bernatik T, Goertz RS. Characterization of focal liver lesions (FLL) with acoustic radiation force impulse (ARFI) elastometry. Ultraschall in der Medizin. 2010;**31**(4):405-409. DOI: 10.1055/s-0029-1245565

[34] Dong Y, Wang WP, Xu Y, Cao J, Mao F, Dietrich CF. Point shear wave speed measurement in differentiating benign and malignant focal liver lesions. Medical Ultrasonography. 2017;**19**(3):259-264. DOI: 10.11152/ mu-1142

[35] Park H, Park JY, Kim DY, Ahn SH, Chon CY, Han KH, et al. Characterization of focal liver masses using acoustic radiation force impulse elastography. World Journal of Gastroenterology. 2013;**19**(2):219-226. DOI: 10.3748/wjg.v19.i2.219

[36] Kim JE, Lee JY, Bae KS, Han JK, Choi BI. Acoustic radiation force impulse elastography for focal hepatic tumors: Usefulness for differentiating

hemangiomas from malignant tumors. Korean Journal of Radiology. 2013;**14**(5):743-753. DOI: 10.3348/kjr.2013.14.5.743

[37] Ghiuchici AM, Sporea I, Dănilă M, Șirli R, Moga T, Bende F, et al. Is there a place for elastography in the diagnosis of hepatocellular carcinoma? Journal of Clinical Medicine. 2021;**10**(8):1710. DOI: 10.3390/jcm10081710

[38] Choong KL, Wong YH, Yeong CH, Gnanasuntharam GK, Goh KL, Yoong BK, et al. Elasticity characterization of liver cancers using shear wave ultrasound elastography: Comparison between hepatocellular carcinoma and liver metastasis. Journal of Diagnostic Medical Sonography. 2017;**33**(6):481-488. DOI: 10.1177/8756479317733713

[39] Gerber L, Fitting D, Srikantharajah K, Weiler N, Kyriakidou G, Bojunga J, et al. Evaluation of 2D- shear wave elastography for characterization of focal liver lesions. Journal of Gastrointestinal and Liver Diseases. 2017;**26**(3):283-290. DOI: 10.15403/jgld.2014.1121.263.dsh

[40] Guo J, Jiang D, Qian Y, Yu J, Gu YJ, Zhou YQ, et al. Differential diagnosis of different types of solid focal liver lesions using two-dimensional shear wave elastography. World Journal of Gastroenterology. 2022;**28**(32):4716-4725. DOI: 10.3748/wjg.v28.i32.4716

[41] Șirli R, Popescu A, Jenssen C, Möller K, Lim A, Dong Y, et al. WFUMB review paper. Incidental findings in otherwise healthy subjects, how to manage: Liver. Cancers (Basel). 2024;**16**(16):2908. DOI: 10.3390/cancers16162908

[42] Zhang HP, Gu JY, Bai M, Li F, Zhou YQ, Du LF. Value of shear wave elastography with maximal elasticity in differentiating benign and malignant solid focal liver lesions. World Journal of Gastroenterology. 2020;**26**(46):7416-7424. DOI: 10.3748/wjg.v26.i46.7416

[43] Shuang-Ming T, Ping Z, Ying Q, Li-Rong C, Ping Z, Rui-Zhen L. Usefulness of acoustic radiation force impulse imaging in the differential diagnosis of benign and malignant liver lesions. Academic Radiology. 2011;**18**(7):810-815. DOI: 10.1016/j.acra.2011.01.026

[44] Cho SH, Lee JY, Han JK, Choi BI. Acoustic radiation force impulse elastography for the evaluation of focal solid hepatic lesions: Preliminary findings. Ultrasound in Medicine & Biology. 2010;**36**(2):202-208. DOI: 10.1016/j.ultrasmedbio.2009.10.009

[45] Ronot M, Di Renzo S, Gregoli B, et al. Characterization of fortuitously discovered focal liver lesions: Additional information provided by shear wave elastography. European Radiology. 2015;**25**:346-358. DOI: 10.1007/s00330-014-3370-z

[46] Singla A, Vishwanath TT, Das SK, Murthy N, Patil V, et al. Evaluation of solid focal liver lesions by shear wave sonoelastography with FNAC correlation. International Journal of Radiology and Imaging Technology. 2020;**6**:064. DOI: 10.23937/2572-3235.1510064

[47] Goya C, Hamidi C, Yavuz A, Hattapoglu S, Uslukaya O, Cetincakmak MG, et al. The role of acoustic radiation force impulse elastography in the differentiation of infectious and neoplastic liver lesions. Ultrasonic Imaging. 2015;**37**(4):312-322. DOI: 10.1177/0161734614566697

[48] Gallotti A, D'Onofrio M, Romanini L, Cantisani V, Pozzi MR.

Acoustic radiation force impulse (ARFI) ultrasound imaging of solid focal liver lesions. European Journal of Radiology. 2012;**81**(3):451-455. DOI: 10.1016/j.ejrad.2010.12.071

[49] Ainora ME, Cerrito L, Liguori A, Mignini I, De Luca A, Galasso L, et al. Multiparametric dynamic ultrasound approach for differential diagnosis of primary liver tumors. International Journal of Molecular Sciences. 2023;**24**(10):8548. DOI: 10.3390/ijms24108548

[50] Serag DM, Ebeid EA, Dessouky B, Omar H. Role of shear wave elastography in characterization of hepatic focal lesions. Egyptian Journal of Radiology and Nuclear Medicine. 2020;**51**:58. DOI: 10.1186/s43055-020-00178-2

[51] Martelletti C, Armandi A, Caviglia GP, Saracco GM, Pellicano R. Elastography for characterization of focal liver lesions: Current evidence and future perspectives. Minerva Gastroenterology (Torino). 2021;**67**(2):196-208. DOI: 10.23736/S2724-5985.20.02747-6

[52] Hasab-Allah M, Salama RM, Marie MS, Mandur AA, Omar H. Utility of point shear wave elastography in characterisation of focal liver lesions. Expert Review of Gastroenterology & Hepatology. 2018;**12**(2):201-207. DOI: 10.1080/17474124.2018.1415144

[53] Sandulescu L, Padureanu V, Dumitrescu C, Braia N, Streba CT, Gheonea DI, et al. A pilot study of real time elastography in the differentiation of focal liver lesions. Current Health Sciences Journal. 2012;**38**(1):32-35

[54] Gheorghe L, Iacob S, Iacob R, Dumbrava M, Becheanu G, Herlea V, et al. Real time elastography - A non-invasive diagnostic method of small hepatocellular carcinoma in cirrhosis.

Journal of Gastrointestinal and Liver Diseases. 2009;**18**(4):439-446

[55] Yuan G, Xie F, Song Y, Li Q, Li R, Hu X, et al. Hepatic tumor stiffness measured by shear wave elastography is prognostic for HCC progression following treatment with anti-PD-1 antibodies plus lenvatinib: A retrospective analysis of two independent cohorts. Frontiers in Immunology. 2022;**13**:868809. DOI: 10.3389/fimmu.2022.868809

[56] Kim B, Kim SS, Cho SW, Cheong JY, Huh J, Kim JK, et al. Liver stiffness in magnetic resonance elastography is prognostic for sorafenib-treated advanced hepatocellular carcinoma. European Radiology. 2021;**31**(4):2507-2517. DOI: 10.1007/s00330-020-07357-9

[57] Lu Q, Ling W, Lu C, Li J, Ma L, Quan J, et al. Hepatocellular carcinoma: Stiffness value and ratio to discriminate malignant from benign focal liver lesions. Radiology. 2015;**275**(3):880-888. DOI: 10.1148/radiol.14131164

[58] Cesario V, Accogli E, Domanico A, Di Lascio FM, Napoleone L, Gasbarrini A, et al. Percutaneous real-time sonoelastography as a non-invasive tool for the characterization of solid focal liver lesions: A prospective study. Digestive and Liver Disease. 2016;**48**(2):182-188. DOI: 10.1016/j.dld.2015.11.005

[59] Abdel-Latif M, Fouda N, Shiha OAG, Rizk AA. Role of shear wave sono-elastography (SWE) in characterization of hepatic focal lesions. Egyptian Journal of Radiology and Nuclear Medicine. 2020;**51**:1-5. DOI: 10.1186/s43055-020-00186-2

[60] Dong Y, Koch J, Alhyari A, Safai Zadeh E, Görg C, Wang WP, et al. Ultrasound elastography

for characterization of focal liver lesions. Zeitschrift für Gastroenterologie. 2023;**61**(4):399-410. DOI: 10.1055/a-1957-7370

[61] Ying L, Lin X, Xie ZL, Tang FY, Hu YP, Shi KQ. Clinical utility of acoustic radiation force impulse imaging for identification of malignant liver lesions: A meta-analysis. European Radiology. 2012;**22**(12):2798-2805. DOI: 10.1007/s00330-012-2540-0

[62] Ma X, Zhan W, Zhang B, Wei B, Wu X, Zhou M, et al. Elastography for the differentiation of benign and malignant liver lesions: A meta-analysis. Tumour Biology. 2014;**35**(5):4489-4497. DOI: 10.1007/s13277-013-1591-4

[63] Jiao Y, Dong F, Wang H, Zhang L, Xu J, Zheng J, et al. Shear wave elastography imaging for detecting malignant lesions of the liver: A systematic review and pooled meta-analysis. Medical Ultrasonography. 2017;**19**(1):16-22. DOI: 10.11152/mu-925

[64] Ruan SM, Huang H, Cheng MQ, Lin MX, Hu HT, Huang Y, et al. Shear-wave elastography combined with contrast-enhanced ultrasound algorithm for noninvasive characterization of focal liver lesions. La Radiologia Medica. 2023;**128**:6-15. DOI: 10.1007/s11547-022-01575-5

[65] Wu JP, Shu R, Zhao YZ, Ma GL, Xue W, He QJ, et al. Comparison of contrast-enhanced ultrasonography with virtual touch tissue quantification in the evaluation of focal liver lesions. Journal of Clinical Ultrasound. 2016;**44**(6):347-353. DOI: 10.1002/jcu.22335

[66] da Silva NPB, Hornung M, Beyer LP, Hackl C, Brunner S, Schlitt HJ, et al. Intraoperative shear wave elastography vs. contrast-enhanced ultrasound for the characterization and differentiation of focal liver lesions to optimize liver tumor surgery. Ultraschall in der Medizin. 2019;**40**(2):205-211. DOI: 10.1055/a-0649-1000

[67] Guo LH, Wang SJ, Xu HX, Sun LP, Zhang YF, Xu JM, et al. Differentiation of benign and malignant focal liver lesions: Value of virtual touch tissue quantification of acoustic radiation force impulse elastography. Medical Oncology. 2015;**32**:68. DOI: 10.1007/s12032-015-0543-9

[68] Youssef AT, ElKayal ES, Abdollah DM, Hassan EA. Is shear wave elastography effective for characterization of hepatic focal lesions. Medical Journal of Cairo University. 2022;**90**(9):1583-1590. DOI: 10.21608/mjcu.2022.271510

[69] Kacała A, Dorochowicz M, Matus I, Puła M, Korbecki A, Sobański M, et al. Hepatic hemangioma: Review of imaging and therapeutic strategies. Medicina (Kaunas, Lithuania). 2024;**60**(3):449. DOI: 10.3390/medicina60030449

[70] Wang Y, Jia L, Wang X, Fu L, Liu J, Qian L. Diagnostic performance of 2-D shear wave elastography for differentiation of hepatoblastoma and hepatic hemangioma in children under 3 years of age. Ultrasound in Medicine & Biology. 2019;**45**(6):1397-1406. DOI: 10.1016/j.ultrasmedbio.2019.02.007

[71] Özmen E, Adaletli I, Kayadibi Y, Emre Ş, Kiliç F, Dervişoğlu S, et al. The impact of share wave elastography in differentiation of hepatic hemangioma from malignant liver tumors in pediatric population. European Journal of Radiology. 2014;**83**(9):1691-1697. DOI: 10.1016/j.ejrad.2014.06.002

[72] Villavicencio Kim J, Wu GY. Focal nodular hyperplasia: A comprehensive review with a particular focus on

pathogenesis and complications. Journal of Clinical and Translational Hepatology. 2024;**12**(2):182-190. DOI: 10.14218/JCTH.2023.00265

[73] Brunel T, Guibal A, Boularan C, Ducerf C, Mabrut JY, Bancel B, et al. Focal nodular hyperplasia and hepatocellular adenoma: The value of shear wave elastography for differential diagnosis. European Journal of Radiology. 2015;**84**(11):2059-2064. DOI: 10.1016/j.ejrad.2015.07.029

[74] Akdoğan E, Yılmaz FG. The role of acoustic radiation force impulse elastography in the differentiation of benign and malignant focal liver masses. The Turkish Journal of Gastroenterology. 2018;**29**(4):456-463. DOI: 10.5152/tjg.2018.11710. Erratum in: Turk J Gastroenterol. 2018;29(6):722. DOI: 10.5152/tjg.2018.191918

[75] Taimr P, Klompenhouwer AJ, Thomeer MGJ, Hansen BE, Ijzermans JNM, de Man RA, et al. Can point shear wave elastography differentiate focal nodular hyperplasia from hepatocellular adenoma. Journal of Clinical Ultrasound. 2018;**46**(6):380-385. DOI: 10.1002/jcu.22603

[76] Nagolu H, Kattoju S, Natesan C, Krishnakumar M, Kumar S. Role of acoustic radiation force impulse elastography in the characterization of focal solid hepatic lesions. Journal of Clinical Imaging Science. 2018;**8**:5. DOI: 10.4103/jcis.JCIS_64_17

[77] Aziz H, Brown ZJ, Eskander MF, Aquina CT, Baghdadi A, Kamel IR, et al. A scoping review of the classification, diagnosis, and management of hepatic adenomas. Journal of Gastrointestinal Surgery. 2022;**26**(4):965-978. DOI: 10.1007/s11605-022-05246-8

[78] Li JW, Ling WW, Lu Q, Lu CL, He D, Luo Y. Liver stiffness and serum alpha-fetoprotein in discriminating small hepatocellular carcinoma from cirrhotic nodule. Ultrasound Quarterly. 2016;**32**(4):319-326. DOI: 10.1097/RUQ.0000000000000244

[79] Jeong JY, Sohn JH, Sohn W, Park CH, Kim TY, Jun DW, et al. Role of shear wave elastography in evaluating the risk of hepatocellular carcinoma in patients with chronic hepatitis B. Gut Liver. 2017;**11**(6):852-859. DOI: 10.5009/gnl16521

[80] Loy LM, Low HM, Choi JY, Rhee H, Wong CF, Tan CH. Variant hepatocellular carcinoma subtypes according to the 2019 WHO classification: An imaging-focused review. AJR. American Journal of Roentgenology. 2022;**219**(2):212-223. DOI: 10.2214/AJR.21.26982

[81] Chen R, Kong W, Gan Y, Ge N, Chen Y, Ding H, et al. Tumour stiffness associated with tumour response to conventional transarterial chemoembolisation for hepatocellular carcinoma: Preliminary findings. Clinical Radiology. 2019;**74**(10):814.e1-814.e7. DOI: 10.1016/j.crad.2019.07.008

[82] Abdelaziz AO, Abdelhalim H, Elsharkawy A, Shousha HI, Abdelmaksoud AH, Soliman ZA, et al. Liver stiffness measurement changes following hepatocellular carcinoma treatment with percutaneous microwave ablation or transarterial chemoembolization: A cohort study. European Journal of Gastroenterology & Hepatology. 2019;**31**(6):685-691. DOI: 10.1097/MEG.0000000000001343

[83] Bo XW, Li XL, Xu HX, Guo le H, Li DD, Liu BJ, et al. 2D shear-wave ultrasound elastography (SWE) evaluation of ablation zone following radiofrequency ablation of liver lesions: Is it more accurate? The British Journal

of Radiology. 2016;**89**(1060):20150852. DOI: 10.1259/bjr.20150852

[84] Varghese T, Techavipoo U, Liu W, Zagzebski JA, Chen Q, Frank G, et al. Elastographic measurement of the area and volume of thermal lesions resulting from radiofrequency ablation: Pathologic correlation. AJR. American Journal of Roentgenology. 2003;**181**:701-707. DOI: 10.2214/ajr.181.3.1810701

[85] Van Vledder MG, Boctor EM, Assumpcao LR, Rivaz H, Foroughi P, Hager GD, et al. Intra-operative ultrasound elasticity imaging for monitoring of hepatic tumour thermal ablation. HPB: The Official Journal of the International Hepato Pancreato Biliary Association. 2010;**12**:717-723. DOI: 10.1111/j.1477257

[86] Lee DH, Lee JM, Yoon JH, Kim YJ, Lee JH, Yu SJ, et al. Liver stiffness measured by two-dimensional shear-wave elastography: Prognostic value after radiofrequency ablation for hepatocellular carcinoma. Liver Cancer. 2018;**7**:65-75. DOI: 10.1159/000484445

[87] Yoon JS, Lee YR, Kweon YO, Tak WY, Jang SY, Park SY, et al. Comparison of acoustic radiation force impulse elastography and transient elastography for prediction of hepatocellular carcinoma recurrence after radiofrequency ablation. European Journal of Gastroenterology & Hepatology. 2018;**30**(10):1230-1236. DOI: 10.1097/MEG.0000000000001170

[88] Praktiknjo M, Krabbe V, Pohlmann A, Sampels M, Jansen C, Meyer C, et al. Evolution of nodule stiffness might predict response to local ablative therapy: A series of patients with hepatocellular carcinoma. PLoS One. 2018;**13**(2):e0192897. DOI: 10.1371/journal.pone.0192897.4.2010.00247.x

[89] Mohebbi A, Mohammadzadeh S, Mohebbi S, Mohammadi A, Tavangar SM. Diagnostic performance of ultrasound elastography in differentiating hepatocellular carcinoma and intrahepatic cholangiocarcinoma: A systematic review and meta-analysis. Abdominal Radiology (New York). 2025;**50**(2):633-645. DOI: 10.1007/s00261-024-04502-6

[90] Gu JH, Zhu L, Jiang TA. Quantitative ultrasound elastography methods in focal liver lesions including hepatocellular carcinoma: From diagnosis to prognosis. Ultrasound Quarterly. 2021;**37**(2):90-96. DOI: 10.1097/RUQ.0000000000000491

[91] Shen Q, Wu W, Wang R, Zhang J, Liu L. A non-invasive predictive model based on multimodality ultrasonography images to differentiate malignant from benign focal liver lesions. Scientific Reports. 2024;**14**(1):23996. DOI: 10.1038/s41598-024-74740-7

[92] Chen CM, Tang YC, Huang SH, Pan KT, Lui KW, Lai YH, et al. Ultrasound tissue scatterer distribution imaging: An adjunctive diagnostic tool for shear wave elastography in characterizing focal liver lesions. Ultrasonics Sonochemistry. 2023;**101**:106716. DOI: 10.1016/j.ultsonch.2023.106716

[93] Dong Y, Qiu Y, Zhang Q, Yang D, Yu L, Wang WP, et al. Preliminary clinical experience with shear wave dispersion imaging for liver viscosity in preoperative diagnosis of focal liver lesions. Zeitschrift für Gastroenterologie. 2020;**58**(9):847-854. DOI: 10.1055/a-1217-7465

[94] Wang K, Yu D, Li G, Wen L, Zhang S. Comparison of the diagnostic performance of shear wave elastography with shear wave dispersion for pre-operative staging of hepatic fibrosis in

patients with hepatocellular carcinoma. European Journal of Radiology. 2022;**154**:110459. DOI: 10.1016/j. ejrad.2022.110459

[95] Schulz M, Wilde AB, Demir M, Müller T, Tacke F, Wree A. Shear wave elastography and shear wave dispersion imaging in primary biliary cholangitis-a pilot study. Quantitative Imaging in Medicine and Surgery. 2022;**12**(2):1235-1242. DOI: 10.21037/qims-21-657

Chapter 4

Practical Applications of EUS Elastography: Evidence and Challenges

Anant Gupta and Sandeep Nijhawan

Abstract

Conventional B-mode endoscopic ultrasound (EUS) imaging may not be sufficient to accurately delineate the lesion's character, and thus, endoscopic ultrasound elastography complements it by visualising the elastic properties of a tissue in focus. Different pathologies, such as inflammation, fibrosis, and malignancy, produce various alterations in the tissue architecture, which brings about a change in its stiffness; this forms the basis of elastography. EUS elastography began with qualitative features, but now the focus is shifting to the use of more objective and reproducible quantitative parameters. EUS-strain elastography (EUS-SE) and EUS-shear wave elastography (EUS-SWE) are being used for diagnosis and characterisation of lesions. Researchers are evaluating and standardising it for usefulness in various diseases such as pancreatic solid lesions, pancreatitis (acute/chronic/autoimmune), lymph nodes, and gastrointestinal and subepithelial lesions.

Keywords: elastography, endoscopic ultrasound, quantitative elastography, strain elastography, pancreatic solid lesion

1. Introduction

Elastography is a method used to measure the stiffness of different tissues [1]. It is available as an integrated software in most endoscopic ultrasound (EUS) machines, using either qualitative or quantitative methods. This technology complements the standard B-mode imaging and permits the analysis of tissue stiffness and changes which can be associated with various pathologies, including malignancy. It has fair accuracy in distinguishing benign from malignant lesions (elastography is more helpful in excluding malignancy rather than for confirming), primarily in the pancreas and lymph nodes. EUS elastography is of use when the area of interest is not accessible by needle/there is a contraindication for needling. It may also reduce the requirement for EUS-guided needling of the suspected lesions, and also helps in guiding the biopsy to areas with the highest suspicion of malignancy.

IntechOpen

2. About EUS elastography

EUS elastography-stiffness measurement is assessed using either a qualitative (strain elastography) or a quantitative method (strain ratio (SR), strain histogram technique, EUS-shear wave measurement (SWM)). Until a few years back, predominantly strain elastography was being used, which uses colour scales to reveal tissue hardness. The disadvantage of this is its inability to quantify tissue hardness and its inability to compare its findings with others. On the contrary, shear-wave velocity (Vs) helps to assess the absolute tissue hardness. Hard tissues show higher Vs. The use of EUS elastography in routine practice is evolving, but it lacks high diagnostic accuracy, especially due to the predominant focus on qualitative methods, which have poor reproducibility and the absence of definitive diagnostic cut-offs.

3. Clinical applications of EUS elastography

All these years, indications have been expanding for the application of EUS-guided elastography. However, two predominant areas of use are for the evaluation of solid pancreatic lesions and enlarged lymph nodes.

3.1 Pancreatic diseases

EUS, now, is an unavoidable modality for the diagnosis and staging of pancreatic lesions. However, the capability of conventional B-mode EUS to differentiate between benign and malignant pancreatic lesions is sub-optimal in certain clinical scenarios [2, 3]. Along with clinical examination, laboratory parameters, and radiologic imaging, EUS elastography use is complementary during the evaluation of pancreatic diseases. Elastography can help us in the diagnosis of pancreatic masses, whereas there is still limited literature regarding its use in pancreatitis.

3.1.1 Assessment of solid pancreatic lesions

Solid pancreatic lesions require accurate assessment, for which EUS elastography is helpful. It was in 2006 that the first study of EUS elastography in pancreatic solid lesions was published [4]. Since then, elastography patterns have been put forward. Even though, these patterns are not pathognomonic, but they are helpful, when there is a clear demarcation from the healthy pancreatic parenchyma (usually of a homogenous green colour).

Qualitative EUS elastography patterns are.

- Homogeneous green pattern (suggests normal pancreatic parenchyma).

- Inflammatory pancreatic lesions have a heterogeneous, mostly green shade with subtle red and yellow colours.

- Malignant lesions appear heterogeneous, blue pattern with small green and red areas (**Figure 1**).

- Pancreatic neuroendocrine malignant lesions typically have a homogeneous blue pattern [5].

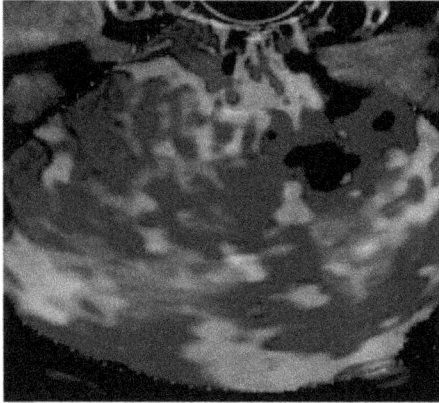

Figure 1.
Qualitative EUS elastography of pancreatic adenocarcinoma shows a predominant blue pattern, and softer (green area) represents a necrotic component.

Different studies have shown different accuracy [6]; there are situations where it is difficult to perform an adequate elastography evaluation – large lesions (>35 mm), lesions at a considerable distance from the transducer, and lesions with fluidic contents (ducts or blood vessels) in the region of interest (ROI). Sophistication and refinement of the software will probably solve these issues.

Using the quantitative assessment, SR of lesion of interest is compared to the SR of the surrounding pancreatic tissue and is apparently much more informative than the conventional qualitative assessment. Higher SR depicts higher chances of malignancy (**Figure 2**) and lower strain histograms than the normal parenchyma [7]. It has been recommended that strain ratio > 10 or strain histogram level < 50 be used to classify lesions as malignant with 100% sensitivity and 92.3% specificity (**Table 1**) [9].

Various meta-analyses have assessed the efficacy of EUS elastography for identifying malignancy in pancreatic lesions. It has been found to have high sensitivity (~95%) but has a low specificity (~70%) (**Tables 2 and 3**) [12–15].

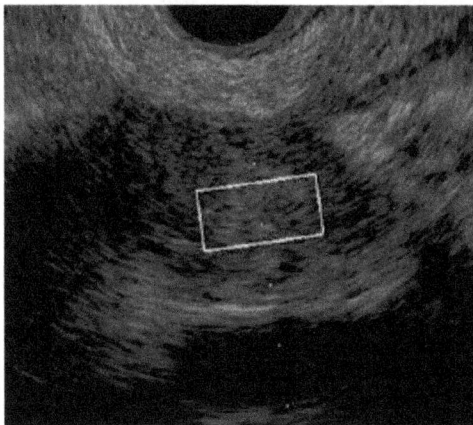

Figure 2.
Pancreatic lesion on which shear-wave elastography has been applied shows shear-wave velocity of 2.6 and kPa (kilopascal) of 20.1.

	Stiffness	Malignant potential
Qualitative Elastography (patterns)		
Blue homogeneous	Hard	Yes
Blue heterogeneous	Hard	Yes
Green Heterogeneous	Intermediate	No
Green Homogenous	Intermediate-soft	No
Heterogeneous green/blue with no predominance	Intermediate-hard	Undetermined
Quantitative Elastography		
Strain Ratio > 10	Hard	Yes
Strain Ratio < 10	Intermediate	No
Strain Histogram >150	Intermediate-soft	No
Strain Histogram 50–150	Intermediate	No
Strain Histogram <50	Hard	Yes

Source: Ref. [8].

Table 1.
Meaning of EUS-guided elastographic evaluation.

Author	Year	Sensitivity (%)	Specificity (%)
Iglesias-Garcia et al.	2009	100	85
Opacic et al	2015	98	50
Okasha et al.	2017	98	77
Kataoka et al.	2021	94	23
Puga-Tejada et al.	2022	94	96

Table 2.
Studies assessing the accuracy of EUS-guided elastography in pancreatic lesions.

Author	Sensitivity (%)	Specificity (%)
Iglesias-Garcia et al. [10] use of qualitative assessment	100	85
Iglesias-Garcia et al. [11] use of quantitative assessment	100	92

Table 3.
Comparing use of qualitative and quantitative assessment.

Smaller lesions are challenging for appropriate sampling due to their size. Due to its high negative predictive value in diagnosing malignancy, EUS elastography is of some help when evaluating small tumours of the pancreas [16]. Using elastography to focus on hard lesions (seen as blue spots) inside the mass-forming chronic pancreatitis (CP) and guide the sampling area is another benefit.

Yamada et al. demonstrated a potential role of elastography in the staging of pancreatic cancer (PC), mainly for vascular compromise [17].

3.1.2 Targeted biopsy

EUS elastography using qualitative application is also useful to detect and focus on harder areas of a particular lesion of interest and helps us to target our sampling needle during EUS-FNA (fine needle aspiration) or fine needle biopsy (FNB). Using this helps us to perform the sampling of the most suitable area, which usually is the blue portion (denoting the presence of a hard lesion; the softer appearing area can probably be necrotic debris) [18]. Overall, there is a 94% diagnostic accuracy of EUS-elastography-guided FNA. It has a 93% sensitivity and 100% specificity for diagnosing malignancy [19]. No large trials comparing EUS-FNA/FNB with and without elastography guide are available. Use of elastography is definitely helpful but not mandatory.

3.1.3 Chronic pancreatitis

Chronic pancreatitis (CP) on routine qualitative EUS elastography shows a predominantly green colour pattern with smaller blue and/or red areas [5]; it is still not pathognomonic for any specific disease. On the other hand, semiquantitative elastography, using histograms or shear waves, helps in the interpretation of the elastography findings.

Higher SR increases the probability of exocrine pancreatic insufficiency and thus elastography also helps in establishing the severity of CP [20]. Using the exocrine pancreatic function tests (ePFTs) as a gold standard, EUS-guided elastography yielded a diagnostic accuracy of 93.4% for CP [21].

Literature shows a positive relationship between pancreatic stiffness (PS) values measured through EUS-SWM value and exocrine/endocrine dysfunction in CP (**Table 4**) [23, 24].

Shear-wave velocity (2.98 m/s) was consistent with CP and the results were significantly higher than those found for normal tissue (1.52 m/s). SWE value had a good linear correlation with the grade of Rosemont classification, whereas the value of strain elastography did not help [23].

Although the diagnostic cut-offs are indistinct, EUS elastography is a promising modality to evaluate pancreatitis. More large-volume research studies will provide clarity and help us improve the diagnostic accuracy.

Age-related changes in the pancreas (appear similar in B-mode to that described for CP) and real CP can also be distinguished using elastography. Studies reveal, despite the age-related hardness in pancreas, on quantitative elastography CP appears harder [25].

Author	Sensitivity (%)	Specificity (%)	Findings
Janssen et al. [5]	65	56	EUS elastography's diagnostic performance in diagnosis CP
Yamashita et al. [22]	83	100	Diagnostic performance of cut-off value of 1.96 pancreatic stiffness in diagnosing CP

Table 4.
Studies on chronic pancreatitis using EUS elastography.

3.1.4 Acute pancreatitis

The application of PS in the evaluation of acute pancreatitis is scarce. No conclusive literature is available to help either in the diagnosis or in the stratification of the severity of acute pancreatitis.

3.1.5 Autoimmune pancreatitis

Autoimmune pancreatitis (AIP) is less common and is underdiagnosed. It has a wide spectrum of radiological features. When there is a focal mass-like lesion, it can be easily confused with pancreatic cancer (PC). This diagnostic dilemma could lead to unnecessary surgery. On elastographic assessment, there is increased hardness in the tumoral area, whereas the entire pancreas appears homogenously stiff in AIP. It thus helps us in differentiating PC from AIP [26].

Normal pancreas appears homogenously green on qualitative elastography, while in AIP, the inflamed pancreatic parenchyma appears mainly green with some smaller areas of red or yellow [5]. However, this is not a consistent feature and is not a reliable pattern to diagnose AIP.

There is no reliable cut-off for diagnosis of AIP, nor there is consensus in differentiating features between focal AIP and PC on quantitative SWE elastography [27].

As of today, elastography is not a mandatory investigation in diagnosing AIP, nor it is a useful stand-alone test to differentiate between PC and focal AIP. However, serial imaging when utilised with EUS elastography and FNB will help us in establishing a diagnosis.

3.2 Lymph nodes

Several researchers have shown the usefulness of EUS-guided elastography in the evaluation of lymph nodes (LN). A green pattern on elastography is 100% likely to be benign (**Figure 3**), whereas a predominant blue pattern (**Figure 3**) is 92% likely to be malignant histology. With mixed patterns on elastography, the likelihood of malignant histology becomes 50% [4, 28–30].

One meta-analysis of seven studies revealed that EUS-guided elastography is an encouraging, non-invasive modality for differentiating high-risk LNs. It will be a useful complementary technique to EUS-guided sampling [31].

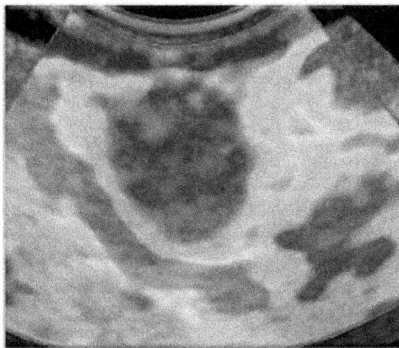

Figure 3.
Quantitative EUS elastography of a lymph node, with a blue predominant pattern, corresponding to a malignant lymph node.

3.3 Gastrointestinal lesions

While evaluating subepithelial lesions, we must differentiate gastrointestinal stromal tumours (GIST) from other mesenchymal lesions such as schwannoma or leiomyoma. Although EUS-guided sampling has demonstrated good accuracy, but sampling small lesions is difficult and, at times, unfruitful [32]. For the diagnosis of such lesions, imaging-based differentiation using EUS elastography might help.

There is no consensus but, according to some researchers, GIST appears as a "hard" tissue when compared to other subepithelial lesions like ectopic pancreas and lipoma [33].

On the other hand, some researchers found it difficult to distinguish GIST from benign leiomyoma [34]. There is a need for further research on whether EUS-guided elastography will be useful in this field.

4. Transrectal EUS elastography

Transrectal EUS elastography is utilised for the diagnosis and assessment of rectal malignancy, inflammatory bowel disease, pelvic floor dyssynergia and prostate malignancy.

Transrectal elastography helps to differentiate between benign and malignant rectal tumours. Quantitative elastography using the SR distinguished between adenomas and adenocarcinomas with a sensitivity of 93%, specificity of 96%, and accuracy of 94% [35, 36].

The rectal wall thickness assessed using strain ratio by EUS elastography has been investigated for evaluation of inflammatory bowel disease and if it reliably helps differentiate Crohn's disease and ulcerative colitis. Higher strain ratios were seen in Chron's disease as compared to controls and ulcerative colitis patients [37].

Elastography is worthier than transrectal EUS alone for establishing the diagnosis of prostatic malignancy, and it increases the accuracy of sampling by focusing on harder areas which have a high degree of malignancy suspicion [38–41].

In pelvic floor dyssynergia, EUS elastography did not show any significant correlation between the patients' assessment, clinical parameters, and the anal sphincter [42, 43].

5. Liver elastography

Liver biopsy is a gold standard technique for the assessment of fibrosis, but it is an invasive method and can have complications. So, gradually, transabdominal ultrasound transient elastography (TUS-TE) came to our rescue, but in patients with ascites or obesity, it may not be reliable. Endoscopic ultrasound elastography is more sensitive than TUS-TE for determining liver fibrosis and detecting liver lesions. EUS elastography assesses more areas of the liver and with better diagnostic efficacy [44].

6. Other indications

EUS-guided elastography may be utilised to evaluate solid adrenal lesions by distinguishing adenomas from metastases. Assessment of liver fibrosis and differentiating benign from malignant liver lesions are probable, possible uses [45].

7. Pitfalls of EUS elastography

No modality is without limitation. The elastographic assessments are observer-dependent due to selection bias for ROI. Secondly, there is endoscopist's inability to control and manage tissue compression, which is another factor. Another limitation is the artefacts caused by other organs (e.g. in smaller spaces like mediastinum, or the presence of cysts, vessels etc) and limited depth of visualisation.

8. Conclusions

EUS-elastography is a risk-free, high-quality tool that complements the findings from B-mode EUS imaging. It is capable of differentiating fibrotic/inflammatory tissues from malignant lesions. It helps to differentiate benign and malignant solid pancreatic lesions with high accuracy, as well as normal pancreas from early CP. The simultaneous use of EUS elastography with FNA and contrast-enhanced EUS is likely to improve the accuracy of the diagnosis [19].

Further research is required to standardise the evaluation method, increase the repeatability and establish definitive values to decide between benign and malignant lesions.

Author details

Anant Gupta[1*] and Sandeep Nijhawan[2]

1 Gastroenterologist, Fortis Escorts Hospital, Jaipur, India

2 Gastroenterologist, Mahatma Gandhi Medical College, Jaipur, India

*Address all correspondence to: dranantg@gmail.com

IntechOpen

References

[1] Tolunay HE, Eroğlu H, Çelik ÖY, Arat Ö, Obut M, Varlı EN, et al. Can placental elasticity predict the time of delivery in cases of threatened preterm labor? The Journal of Obstetrics and Gynaecology Research. 2021;**47**:606-612. DOI: 10.1111/jog.14570

[2] Iglesias-García J, Lindkvist B, Lariño-Noia J, Domínguez-Muñoz JE. The role of EUS in relation to other imaging modalities in the differential diagnosis between mass forming chronic pancreatitis, autoimmune pancreatitis and ductal pancreatic adenocarcinoma. Revista Española de Enfermedades Digestivas. 2012;**104**:315-321

[3] van Huijgevoort NCM, Del Chiaro M, Wolfgang CL, van Hooft JE, Besselink MG. Diagnosis and management of pancreatic cystic neoplasms: Current evidence and guidelines. Nature Reviews. Gastroenterology and Hepatology. 2019;**16**:676-689

[4] Giovannini M, Hookey LC, Bories E, Pesenti C, Monges G, Delpero JR. Endoscopic ultrasound elastography: The first step towards virtual biopsy? Preliminary results in 49 patients. Endoscopy. 2006;**38**:344-348

[5] Janssen J, Schlörer E, Greiner L. EUS elastography of the pancreas: Feasibility and pattern description of the normal pancreas, chronic pancreatitis, and focal pancreatic lesions. Gastrointestinal Endoscopy. 2007;**65**:971-978. DOI: 10.1016/j.gie.2006.12.057

[6] Iglesias-Garcia J, Larino-Noia J, Abdulkader I, Forteza J, Dominguez-Munoz JE. EUS elastography for the characterization of solid pancreatic masses. Gastrointestinal Endoscopy. 2009;**70**:1101-1108

[7] Ying L, Lin X, Xie ZL, Hu YP, Tang KF, Shi KQ. Clinical utility of endoscopic ultrasound elastography for identification of malignant pancreatic masses: A meta-analysis. Journal of Gastroenterology and Hepatology. 2013;**28**:1434-1443. DOI: 10.1111/jgh.12292

[8] Iglesias-Garcia J, de la Iglesia-Garcia D, Lariño-Noia J, Dominguez-Muñoz JE. Endoscopic ultrasound (EUS) guided elastography. Diagnostics. 2023;**13**:1686. DOI: 10.3390/diagnostics13101686

[9] Iglesias-Garcia J, Lindkvist B, Lariño-Noia J, Abdulkader-Nallib I, Dominguez-Muñoz JE. Differential diagnosis of solid pancreatic masses: Contrast-enhanced harmonic (CEH-EUS), quantitative-elastography (QE-EUS), or both? United European Gastroenterology Journal. 2017;**5**:236-246

[10] Iglesias Garcia J, Larino Noia J, Dominguez Munoz JE. Endoscopic ultrasound in the diagnosis and staging of pancreatic cancer. Revista Espanola De Enfermedades Digestivas [Online]. 2009;**101**(9):631-638. ISSN 1130-0108

[11] Iglesias-Garcia J, Larino-Noia J, Abdulkader I, Forteza J, Dominguez-Munoz JE. Quantitative endoscopic ultrasound elastography: An accurate method for the differentiation of solid pancreatic masses. Gastroenterology. 2010;**139**(4):1172-1180. DOI: 10.1053/j.gastro.2010.06.059. Epub 2010 Jun 27

[12] Hu DM, Gong TT, Zhu Q. Endoscopic ultrasound elastography for differential diagnosis of pancreatic masses: A meta-analysis. Digestive Diseases and Sciences. 2013;**58**:1125-1131

[13] Lu Y, Chen L, Li C, Chen H, Chen J. Diagnostic utility of endoscopic ultrasonography-elastography in the evaluation of solid pancreatic masses: A meta-analysis and systematic review. Medical Ultrasonography. 2017;**19**:150-158

[14] Mei M, Ni J, Liu D, Jin P, Sun L. EUS elastography for diagnosis of solid pancreatic masses: A meta-analysis. Gastrointestinal Endoscopy. 2013;**77**:578-589

[15] Zhang B, Zhu F, Li P, Yu S, Zhao Y, Li M. Endoscopic ultrasound elastography in the diagnosis of pancreatic masses: A meta-analysis. Pancreatology. 2018;**18**:833-840

[16] Ignee A, Jenssen C, Arcidiacono PG, Hocke M, Möller K, Saftoiu A, et al. Endoscopic ultrasound elastography of small solid pancreatic lesions: A multicenter study. Endoscopy. 2018;**50**:1071-1079

[17] Yamada K, Kawashima H, Ohno E, Ishikawa T, Tanaka H, Nakamura M, et al. Diagnosis of vascular invasion in pancreatic ductal adenocarcinoma using endoscopic ultrasound elastography. BMC Gastroenterology. 2020;**20**:81

[18] Jafri M, Sachdev AH, Khanna L, Gress FG. The role of real time endoscopic ultrasound guided elastography for targeting EUS-FNA of suspicious pancreatic masses: A review of the literature and a single center experience. Journal of the Pancreas: JOP. 2016;**17**:516-524

[19] Facciorusso A, Martina M, Buccino RV, Nacchiero MC, Muscatiello N. Diagnostic accuracy of fine-needle aspiration of solid pancreatic lesions guided by endoscopic ultrasound elastography. Annals of Gastroenterology. 2018;**31**:513-518. DOI: 10.20524/aog.2018.0271

[20] Dominguez-Muñoz JE, Iglesias-Garcia J, Castiñeira Alvariño M, Luaces Regueira M, Lariño-Noia J. EUS elastography to predict pancreatic exocrine insufficiency in patients with chronic pancreatitis. Gastrointestinal Endoscopy. 2015;**81**:136-142

[21] Iglesias-Garcia J, Lariño-Noia J, Nieto Bsn L, Alvarez-Castro A, Lojo S, Leal S, et al. Pancreatic Elastography predicts endoscopic secretin-pancreatic function test result in patients with early changes of chronic pancreatitis: A prospective, cross-sectional, observational study. American Journal of Gastroenterology. 2022;**117**:1264-1268

[22] Yamashita Y, Tanioka K, Kawaji Y, Tamura T, Nuta J, Hatamaru K, et al. Endoscopic ultrasonography shear wave as a predictive factor of endocrine/exocrine dysfunction in chronic pancreatitis. Journal of Gastroenterology and Hepatology. 2021;**36**:391-396. DOI: 10.1111/jgh.15137

[23] Yamashita Y, Yamazaki H, Shimokawa T, Kawaji Y, Tamumra T, Hatamaru K, et al. Shear-wave versus strain elastography in endoscopic ultrasound for the diagnosis of chronic pancreatitis. Pancreatology. 2023;**23**:35-41

[24] Domínguez-Muñoz JE, Alvarez-Castro A, Lariño-Noia J, Nieto L, Iglesias-García J. Endoscopic ultrasonography of the pancreas as an indirect method to predict pancreatic exocrine insufficiency in patients with chronic pancreatitis. Pancreas. 2012;**41**:724-728. DOI: 10.1097/MPA.0b013e31823b5978

[25] Janssen J, Papavassiliou I. Effect of aging and diffuse chronic

pancreatitis on pancreas elasticity evaluated using semiquantitative EUS elastography. Ultraschall in der Medizin. 2014;**35**:253-258

[26] Conti CB, Cereatti F, Drago A, Grassia R. Focal autoimmune pancreatitis: A simple flow chart for a challenging diagnosis. Ultrasound International Open. 2020;**6**:E67-E75. DOI: 10.1055/a-1323-4906

[27] Ishikawa T, Kawashima H, Ohno E, Tanaka H, Maeda K, Sawada T, et al. Usefulness of endoscopic ultrasound elastography combined with the strain ratio in the estimation of treatment effect in autoimmune pancreatitis. Pancreas. 2020;**49**:e21-e22. DOI: 10.1097/MPA.0000000000001481

[28] Giovannini M, Thomas B, Erwan B, Christian P, Fabrice C, Benjamin E, et al. Endoscopic ultrasound elastography for evaluation of lymph nodes and pancreatic masses: A multicenter study. World Journal of Gastroenterology. 2009;**15**:1587-1593

[29] Dietrich CF, Jenssen C, Arcidiacono PG, Cui XW, Giovannini M, Hocke M, et al. Endoscopic ultrasound: Elastographic lymph node evaluation. Endoscopic Ultrasound. 2015;**4**:176-190

[30] Janssen J, Dietrich CF, Will U, Greiner L. Endosonographic elastography in the diagnosis of mediastinal lymph nodes. Endoscopy. 2007;**39**:952-957

[31] Xu W, Shi J, Zeng X, Li X, Xie WF, Guo J, et al. EUS elastography for the differentiation of benign and malignant lymph nodes: A meta-analysis. Gastrointestinal Endoscopy. 2011;**74**:1001-1009

[32] Akahoshi K, Oya M, Koga T, Koga H, Motomura Y, Kubokawa M, et al. Clinical usefulness of endoscopic ultrasound-guided fine needle aspiration for gastric subepithelial lesions smaller than 2 cm. Journal of Gastrointestinal and Liver Diseases. 2014;**23**:405-412

[33] Tsuji Y, Kusano C, Gotoda T, Itokawa F, Fukuzawa M, Sofuni A, et al. Diagnostic potential of endoscopic ultrasonography-elastography for gastric submucosal tumors: A pilot study. Digestive Endoscopy. 2016;**28**:173-178

[34] Ignee A, Jenssen C, Hocke M, Dong Y, Wang WP, Cui XW, et al. Contrast-enhanced (endoscopic) ultrasound and endoscopic ultrasound elastography in gastrointestinal stromal tumors. Endoscopic Ultrasound. 2017;**6**:55-60

[35] Waage JER, Rafaelsen SR, Borley NR, Havre RF, Gubberud ET, Leh S, et al. Strain Elastography evaluation of rectal tumors: Inter- and Intraobserver reproducibility. Ultraschall in der Medizin. 2015;**36**:611-617

[36] Waage JER, Leh S, Røsler C, Pfeffer F, Bach SP, Havre RF, et al. Endorectal ultrasonography, strain elastography and MRI differentiation of rectal adenomas and adenocarcinomas. Colorectal Disease. 2015;**17**:124-131

[37] Rustemovic N, Cukovic-Cavka S, Brinar M, Radić D, Opacic M, Ostojic R, et al. A pilot study of transrectal endoscopic ultrasound elastography in inflammatory bowel disease. BMC Gastroenterology. 2011;**11**:113

[38] Kamoi K, Okihara K, Ochiai A, Ukimura O, Mizutani Y, Kawauchi A, et al. The utility of transrectal real-time elastography in the diagnosis of prostate cancer. Ultrasound in Medicine and Biology. 2008;**34**:1025-1032

[39] Kapoor A, Kapoor A, Mahajan G, Sidhu BS. Real-time elastography in the

detection of prostate cancer in patients with raised PSA level. Ultrasound in Medicine and Biology. 2011;37:1374-1381

[40] Giurgiu CR, Manea C, Crişan N, Bungărdean C, Coman I, Dudea SM. Real-time sonoelastography in the diagnosis of prostate cancer. Medical Ultrasonography. 2011;13:5-9

[41] Miyagawa T, Tsutsumi M, Matsumura T, Kawazoe N, Ishikawa S, Shimokama T, et al. Real-time elastography for the diagnosis of prostate cancer: Evaluation of elastographic moving images. Japanese Journal of Clinical Oncology. 2009;39:394-398

[42] Rimbaş M, Gheonea DI, Săndulescu L, Săftoiu A, Vilmann P, Ciurea T. EUS Elastography in evaluating chronic liver disease. Why not from Inside? Current Health Sciences Journal. 2009;35:225-227

[43] Allgayer H, Ignee A, Dietrich CF. Endosonographic elastography of the anal sphincter in patients with fecal incontinence. Scandinavian Journal of Gastroenterology. 2010;45:30-38

[44] Oeda S, Tanaka K, Oshima A, Matsumoto Y, Sueoka E, Takahashi H. Diagnostic accuracy of FibroScan and factors affecting measurements. Diagnostics (Basel). 2020;10(11):940. DOI: 10.3390/diagnostics10110940

[45] Iglesias García J, Lariño Noia J, Souto R, Alvarez Castro A, Cigarrán B, Domínguez Muñoz JE. Endoscopic ultrasound (EUS) elastography of the liver. Revista Española de Enfermedades Digestivas. 2009;101:717-719

Chapter 5

Bioethical Implications of Elastrography

Hector Fabio Restrepo-Guerrero

Abstract

Elastography, as an advanced diagnostic tool, raises various bioethical challenges in clinical practice. Key issues include safeguarding patient data privacy, as this technology generates sensitive information about tissue elasticity. Additionally, equitable access to this technology raises concerns, particularly in regions with fewer resources. The increasing use of artificial intelligence in interpreting results also introduces ethical dilemmas, such as transparency in the algorithms used and accountability in case of errors. Ensuring that patients provide informed consent, fully understanding how their data will be used and the associated risks, is crucial. Addressing these ethical considerations is essential to ensure that elastography is applied fairly and responsibly.

Keywords: elastography, bioethics, magnetic resonance imaging, doppler ultrasound, medical technology

1. Introduction

Elastography is an advanced medical imaging technique that assesses the elasticity and stiffness of soft tissues, providing additional information that complements images obtained by conventional methods such as ultrasound and Magnetic Resonance Imaging (MRI). This methodology has established itself as an essential tool in the diagnosis of various pathologies, including liver diseases, breast, thyroid, and prostate cancer, among others. The ability to differentiate normal from pathological tissues by measuring their biomechanical properties allows for earlier and more accurate detection of abnormalities, thereby improving clinical outcomes [1–3].

Elastography was developed in the 1990s as an extension of conventional ultrasound, with the aim of measuring the elasticity of tissues by applying mechanical or acoustic waves. Since its inception, the technique has undergone significant technological advances that have expanded its clinical applications and improved its accuracy and reliability. The introduction of modalities such as magnetic resonance elastography and three-dimensional elastography has allowed for a more detailed and specific evaluation of various medical conditions, positioning elastography as an indispensable tool in modern diagnosis [4–6].

Bioethics is a discipline that focuses on the ethical aspects of medical practice and scientific research, based on fundamental principles such as autonomy, beneficence, nonmaleficence, and justice. These principles guide decision-making in health care, ensuring that patients' rights and well-being are respected and protected. In the context of emerging technologies, such as elastography, bioethics plays a crucial role in assessing the ethical implications of their use and development [7–9].

The incorporation of new medical technologies such as elastography raises a series of bioethical considerations that must be addressed to ensure their responsible and equitable use. These considerations include risk-benefit assessment, equitable access to technology, privacy, and confidentiality of patient data, as well as informed consent. Analyzing elastography from a bioethical perspective makes it possible to identify and mitigate possible ethical dilemmas, promoting a medical practice that respects the fundamental values and rights of patients [7, 10].

The adoption of advanced technologies such as elastography must be guided not only by their clinical efficacy, but also by a strong ethical framework that ensures their fair and responsible implementation. Without proper bioethical assessment, there is a risk that these technologies will exacerbate inequalities in access to health-care or compromise patient autonomy. Therefore, the integration of bioethics into the evaluation of elastography is essential to ensure that its use benefits society as a whole and respects individual rights [7, 11, 12].

The analysis of elastography from a bioethical perspective is fundamental to addressing the ethical challenges that arise with its use and development. This approach not only ensures that ethical principles are respected in clinical practice but also contributes to the development of policies and regulations that promote equitable and safe use of technology. In addition, by considering the ethical implica-tions of elastography, healthcare professionals can make more informed and ethically responsible decisions, thereby improving the quality of healthcare and patients' trust in healthcare services [7, 13, 14].

2. Bioethics in diagnostic imaging techniques

2.1 Introduction to bioethical principles in the use of medical technologies

The use of medical technologies such as elastography in clinical diagnosis requires the careful application of bioethical principles to ensure that patients' well-being and rights are protected. The four fundamental principles of bioethics—autonomy, beneficence, nonmaleficence, and justice—provide a solid framework to guide responsible and equitable medical practice. In the case of emerging technologies, such as diagnostic imaging methods, these principles become even more important, as rapid technological evolution can present complex ethical dilemmas [7, 8, 11].

2.2 Autonomy in diagnostic procedures

The principle of autonomy refers to the patient's right to make informed decisions about their own treatment, including accepting or rejecting diagnostic procedures such as elastography. In this context, it is essential that clinicians provide clear and comprehensive information about the benefits, risks, and alternatives avail-able, allowing patients to make decisions based on a proper understanding of their options. The introduction of new technologies may challenge this principle, as some patients might feel pressured to accept advanced technological procedures without fully understanding their implications [7, 15, 16].

2.3 Beneficence and non-maleficence in diagnostic imaging

The principle of beneficence requires that health professionals act in the best interest of the patient, seeking to maximize the benefits of diagnosis and treatment. On the other hand, the principle of non-maleficence requires doctors to avoid causing harm. In the case of elastography, these principles need to be carefully balanced, as although the technology can offer significant benefits in the early detection of diseases, its misuse or unjustified use could lead to misdiagnosis, unnecessary anxiety, or inappropriate treatments. In addition, incorrect interpretation of images can have adverse consequences for the patient, highlighting the importance of proper training of physicians using these technologies [8, 17, 18].

2.4 Informed consent and new technologies

Informed consent is a critical component of respecting patient autonomy and is particularly relevant in the use of advanced technologies such as elastography. This process involves not only obtaining the patient's consent but also the obligation to explain in detail how the technology works, what its possible outcomes are, and what other diagnostic options are available. Since many patients may not be familiar with emerging technologies, clinicians must be especially careful to ensure that the information provided is understandable and accessible [10, 19, 20].

2.5 Justice and equity in access to technology

The principle of justice in bioethics refers to the equitable distribution of health resources, ensuring that all patients have access to the same diagnostic and therapeutic opportunities. In the case of elastography, a relatively expensive and highly specialized technology, ethical questions arise about equity in its access. Patients in rural or under-resourced areas might not have access to these advanced technologies, raising ethical dilemmas in terms of distributive justice. Health systems must work to minimize these disparities and ensure that technology benefits as many patients as possible, regardless of their geographic location or economic situation [11, 21, 22].

2.6 Ethical responsibility in the interpretation and communication of results

An important part of ethical practice in diagnostic imaging involves the proper interpretation of results and the effective communication of the results to patients. In the case of elastography, this is especially relevant due to the technical complexity of the images generated and the possible difficulty of explaining their implications to patients. Clinicians need to ensure that patients understand their test results clearly and accurately without raising unnecessary alarms or minimizing potential risks. In addition, they must provide recommendations based on evidence and in the best interest of the patient, which reinforces the principle of beneficence [16, 20, 23].

3. Specific bioethical implications of elastography

3.1 Autonomy: Making informed decisions in the use of elastography

The principle of autonomy in bioethics emphasizes the right of patients to make informed decisions about their own medical care. In the context of elastography, a relatively new and highly specialized technique, it is critical that patients understand not only the purpose of the examination, but also the associated benefits, limitations, and potential risks. Physicians have an obligation to clearly communicate these aspects, allowing patients to actively participate in decision-making about their diagnosis and treatment. However, the technical complexity of elastography can pose a challenge in ensuring that the patient fully understands the information provided. It is therefore essential that health professionals receive adequate training to transmit this information in an accessible and understandable way [7, 16].

The patient's autonomy is also influenced by the context in which the elastography is performed. In some cases, the limited availability of diagnostic alternatives could pressure patients to accept this technique without a full understanding of its implications. This scenario poses ethical dilemmas, as patients could feel compelled to follow medical advice without being able to fully exercise their autonomy. Consequently, it is crucial that the informed consent process is thorough and that the patient's individual preferences are respected, even when there are technological or access limitations [8, 20].

3.2 Beneficence: Maximizing benefits in elastography

The principle of beneficence requires health professionals to act in the best interests of the patient, promoting interventions that maximize clinical benefits. In the case of elastography, this principle is manifested in the ability of this technology to detect diseases non-invasively and with high accuracy, reducing the need for biopsies or more aggressive procedures. This technique has proven particularly useful in the evaluation of liver fibrosis, breast cancer, and other diseases, improving clinical outcomes and contributing to more effective therapeutic decision-making [2, 3, 7].

However, charity also requires a critical evaluation of when it is appropriate to use elastography. While the technology can offer great benefits, its use indiscriminately or in patients for whom it is not indicated could result in unnecessary expenses or misdiagnoses. Therefore, clinicians must carefully balance the potential benefits with the risks and limitations, ensuring that elastography is used appropriately and for the benefit of the patient. In this sense, continuous training and updating of medical knowledge are essential to ensure that professionals can apply elastography ethically and effectively [3, 18, 23].

3.3 Non-maleficence: Avoiding potential harm in diagnosis

The principle of non-maleficence refers to the obligation of health professionals to avoid causing harm to patients. Although elastography is a non-invasive and generally safe technique, it is important to consider that no medical procedure is without risk. Incorrect interpretation of images or overreliance on this technology can lead to misdiagnosis, which could lead to inadequate treatments or delays in necessary interventions. This highlights the importance of physicians being properly trained in interpreting elastography images and integrating their results with other diagnostic methods [7, 5, 17].

In addition, overuse of diagnostic technologies such as elastography can lead to unnecessary anxiety in patients, especially if results are inconclusive or uncertain findings are discovered that require prolonged follow-up. To avoid this, practitioners need to be transparent in communicating the limits and possibilities of elastography, ensuring that patients understand that it is not always possible to get definitive answers through this technique. This minimizes the risk of psychological harm and ensures a more positive experience for patients [18, 20].

3.4 Justice: Equitable access to elastography

The principle of justice in bioethics focuses on the equitable distribution of resources and medical care. In the context of elastography, an advanced technology that is not yet widely available in all regions, significant ethical challenges related to equity in access arise. Patients in rural areas or in developing countries may not have access to this technology, creating significant disparities in the diagnosis and treatment of diseases. This lack of access raises a question of distributive justice, as patients who could benefit from elastography are not always able to access it due to geographical or economic limitations [11, 21, 22].

To address this ethical dilemma, health systems and regulatory authorities should consider strategies to expand access to elastography, such as grants for health centers in underserved areas or policies that promote the acquisition of this technology in public hospitals. It is also crucial that technological advances are accompanied by efforts to reduce the economic barriers that prevent its equitable use, ensuring that the benefits of elastography are available to all patients, regardless of their location or socioeconomic status [11, 22].

3.5 Informed consent in elastography: A bioethical challenge

Informed consent is a crucial process that respects patient autonomy, but it can become particularly challenging in the context of technologies such as

Bioethical challenge	Description	Potential impact	Proposed solution
Data Privacy	Elastography generates sensitive images and data about the patient.	Exposure to privacy breaches or data misuse.	Implement security protocols and data encryption.
Equity in access	Inequality in access to technology in different regions.	Patients in rural or low-resource areas may be left without access.	Health policies that promote equitable access.
Algorithmic Accountability	Reliance on AI for interpretation of elastography results.	Dehumanization in diagnosis and automated errors.	Maintain human supervision in decision-making.
Validity of the results	Lack of standardization in procedures can affect validity.	Unreliable results can affect diagnosis and treatment.	Develop international standards and continuous validation.
Informed consent	Patients need to understand how the data obtained is used.	Possible lack of transparency and violation of patients' rights.	Ensure clear communication and obtain informed consent.

Source: Authors.

Table 1.
Bioethical challenges of elastography.

elastography, which are complex and relatively new. The technical nature of elastography and the unfamiliarity of many patients with this type of diagnosis can make it difficult to understand, making the informed consent process more complicated. Healthcare professionals must be able to explain the procedure, its benefits, and its risks in a way that is clear and accessible, adapting to each patient's level of understanding (**Table 1**) [16, 19, 20].

It is important for doctors to not only provide technical information but also to ensure that patients understand how elastography results could affect their treatment and prognosis. In addition, the use of emerging technologies such as elastography in clinical research raises the need for even more rigorous informed consent, where patients must be aware that the technology could be in the experimental phase and that the results are not always conclusive. In this regard, health institutions must provide clear and ethical guidelines to ensure that informed consent is given appropriately and ethically [10].

4. Challenges and future perspectives in elastography from bioethics

4.1 The balance between technological innovation and ethical responsibility

Elastography, as an emerging technology, faces the challenge of balancing its growth and development with a solid foundation of ethical responsibility. As technology advances and its clinical applications expand, it is essential that developers, researchers, and healthcare professionals consider not only the potential medical benefit but also the ethical implications of its use. This balance requires constant vigilance to ensure that elastography is used fairly, responsibly, and in line with fundamental ethical principles, such as beneficence, non-maleficence, autonomy, and justice [7, 11].

Technological progress always carries potential risks, and in the case of elastography, this includes the possibility of errors in the interpretation of results, excessive or inappropriate use of technology, and unequal access to the benefits of this tool. Therefore, there is a need for clear ethical guidelines to be implemented that regulate both research and clinical practice related to elastography. The establishment of clinical ethics committees and ongoing bioethics training for professionals using these technologies are key steps in ensuring that the development of elastography follows an appropriate ethical course [10, 22].

4.2 Challenges in equity and access to elastography

One of the most significant challenges in the expansion of elastography is to ensure equitable access to this technology. Disparities in health care, especially in less developed regions or among marginalized populations, represent a considerable obstacle to the fair implementation of elastography. In many developing countries, access to advanced technologies such as elastography is limited, leading to inequalities in the diagnosis and treatment of diseases that could benefit greatly from this tool [21, 24].

To address this challenge, it is critical that governments, international organizations, and health systems work together to foster policies that promote equitable accessibility to elastography. This may involve subsidies, training programs for medical personnel in remote regions, and the acquisition of technological equipment in public health centers. In the long term, developing more accessible and cost-effective versions of elastography could also help bridge the gap in access to this technology [22].

4.3 The challenge of ethical use in clinical research

Research with emerging medical technologies, such as elastography, raises complex ethical questions, particularly as it pertains to experimentation on human subjects. While elastography has enormous potential, its experimental use must be rigorously regulated to avoid situations where participants are exposed to unnecessary risks. In this regard, informed consent remains a central concern, and it must be ensured that participants understand the risks and benefits of their participation in clinical studies [16, 25].

Clinical trials must also ensure that the data obtained benefit society as a whole and not just the institutions that fund the research. This implies full transparency in the results of studies and a commitment to share findings, both positive and negative, with the scientific community and the general public. The ethics of elastography research should also address access to treatments derived from research findings, ensuring that the benefits of the technology are available to all patients, regardless of socioeconomic or geographic status [23, 24].

4.4 Responsibility for the training and use of elastography

Another bioethical challenge in the use of elastography lies in the training and responsibility of health professionals. Since elastography is a complex and constantly evolving technology, professionals who employ it must receive adequate and continuous training to ensure that its use is carried out competently and ethically. Incorrect interpretation of images or misuse of technology could have detrimental consequences for patients, underscoring the importance of professional competence in this area [18].

In addition, regulatory bodies should establish training and certification standards for professionals who use elastography in clinical practice. This responsibility also extends to medical and educational institutions, which must ensure that teaching about elastography includes not only technical aspects, but also ethical considerations related to its use, interpretation, and communication of results. This will help prevent medical errors and ensure that patients receive care based on the highest standards of medical ethics [20].

4.5 Future perspectives in the bioethical regulation of elastography

As elastography continues to develop, so will the need for robust bioethical regulation. In the future, ethics committees are expected to play an increasingly important role in reviewing and regulating the use of emerging technologies, ensuring that new applications of elastography are implemented fairly and ethically. This could include the creation of specific ethical frameworks for the assessment of new medical technologies and the establishment of international guidelines that promote equity in access to and use of elastography [26].

Future prospects also include the development of artificial intelligence (AI) elastography to improve its accuracy and reduce the margin for human error. Nonetheless, this raises new bioethical concerns, especially with regard to data privacy and transparency in automated clinical decision-making. It will be essential that the development of AI in elastography is carried out under strict ethical supervision to ensure that its implementation respects the rights of patients and maintains high standards of justice, autonomy, and fairness [27].

4.6 The role of bioethics in the social acceptance of elastography

Finally, the social acceptance of elastography also depends to a large extent on how its ethical aspects are handled. Patients and the general public should feel confident that medical technologies that affect their health are developed and used ethically and responsibly. Transparency in research processes, equitable access to technological benefits, and ensuring that patients can make informed decisions are key factors that will influence public acceptance and trust in elastography [19].

Educational campaigns that inform the public about the benefits and limitations of elastography, along with the implementation of clear policies that protect patients and ensure responsible use of the technology, will contribute to social acceptance. Ultimately, the role of bioethics is to ensure that medical innovations, such as elastography, are integrated into clinical practice in ways that respect and promote fundamental ethical principles [7].

5. Clinical applications of elastography and bioethical dilemmas

5.1 The use of elastography in clinical practice

Elastography has emerged as a crucial tool in various medical specialties, especially in areas such as hepatology, oncology, and rheumatology. In hepatology, elastography is primarily used for the evaluation of liver fibrosis, providing a non-invasive method for the detection and monitoring of chronic liver disease. In oncology, its ability to differentiate soft tissues based on stiffness has facilitated the early identification of tumors, especially in breast, thyroid, and prostate cancers. In rheumatology, it is used to evaluate soft tissue conditions and inflammation in autoimmune diseases such as rheumatoid arthritis [3, 28, 29].

Despite advances in these areas, the widespread use of elastography in clinical practice poses ethical challenges related to access, equity, and interpretation of results. The availability of technology in clinical settings depends on economic and logistical factors, which can lead to inequalities in its use. In addition, healthcare professionals must be properly trained to interpret elastography results, as incorrect interpretation of these data can lead to misdiagnosis, resulting in potential harm to patients [22, 26].

5.2 Ethical dilemmas in the early detection of diseases

One of the greatest benefits of elastography is its ability to detect certain diseases early, which can significantly improve clinical outcomes. However, this advantage also raises important ethical dilemmas. Early detection of diseases such as cancer can raise concerns about overdiagnosis, which occurs when abnormalities are identified that may not cause significant clinical harm throughout the patient's lifetime. This type of overdiagnosis can lead to unnecessary treatments, increasing the associated risks and costs, with no real benefit to the patient.

This problem is closely linked to the issue of informed consent. Patients should understand not only the potential benefits of elastography, but also the associated

risks, including false positives and overdiagnosis. In addition, health care professionals have a responsibility to discuss with patients the uncertainty that may accompany
elastography findings and treatment options, so that patients can make well-informed
decisions about their health [19].

5.3 Equity in access to advanced technologies

Inequity in access to advanced technologies is a persistent challenge in modern
medicine. Elastography, as a diagnostic technology tool, is more widely available in
advanced medical centers, while populations in rural or low-income areas may have
limited access to this technology. This unequal access raises bioethical questions, as
people with fewer resources or who live in geographically isolated areas might not
benefit from the advantages offered by elastography, perpetuating inequalities in
health care [21, 24].

To address this issue, it is critical that public health policies promote the expansion
of access to elastography, ensuring that it is not a technology reserved only for those
with greater economic resources. This may involve investments in health infrastructure in less developed regions and training programs for health professionals working
in these areas. This ensures that the benefits of elastography are equitably accessible
to the entire population [22].

5.4 The role of elastography in personalized medicine

Elastography has the potential to be a key tool in personalized medicine, allowing
for a more precise and tailored approach to the diagnosis and treatment of patients.
For example, in oncology, elastography can help identify the specific location and
characteristics of a tumor, allowing for more targeted and less invasive treatments.
However, the use of this advanced technology also poses ethical challenges related to
the personalization of treatments and equity in their application [2].

Access to personalized medicine, including elastography, is generally tied to
the availability of resources, which can leave certain populations at a disadvantage.
In addition, personalization of treatments based on elastography findings should
be handled carefully to avoid overuse or inappropriate use of expensive therapies,
which might not be warranted in all patients. Healthcare professionals must balance
the accuracy offered by elastography with the principles of justice and equity in
healthcare, ensuring that all patients receive appropriate treatment without creating
unnecessary disparities [11].

5.5 Ethical considerations in the management of diagnostic information

The use of elastography also raises questions related to privacy and the handling of diagnostic information. As technology evolves, elastography is expected
to integrate with other AI-based diagnostic tools, which could make it easier to
store and analyze large amounts of medical data. However, the ethical handling of
this data is crucial to ensure that patient privacy is protected and that data is not
misused [27].

Medical ethics committees should develop clear guidelines for handling information
obtained through elastography, ensuring that data is used only for medical purposes
and that patients have full control over how their information is used. In addition, concerns about potential discrimination based on diagnostic results need to be addressed,

as identifying certain characteristics or predispositions using elastography could lead to misuse of this information in areas such as insurance or employment [26].

In the use of elastography, both the operator and the physician have a crucial ethical responsibility to ensure that patients understand that the values obtained are not absolute. It is essential that healthcare professionals explain that results may vary due to factors such as the technique employed, patient conditions, and operator experience. In methods such as transient elastography, interobserver and intraobserver variability has been observed to be as high as 20%, meaning that values can change between measurements made by different operators or even by the same operator at different times. This inherent variability must be communicated clearly and honestly so that patients do not interpret the results as definitive or accurate with no margin for error.

Transparency in this process not only promotes a relationship of trust between the patient and the professional but is also key to informed consent. Patients should understand that elastography, while a powerful tool, has limitations that can influence the interpretation of its results. By highlighting these points, physicians and operators can help avoid misunderstandings and unrealistic expectations, ensuring that clinical decisions are made with full awareness of possible variations. This ethical responsibility strengthens patient-centered care and avoids overreliance on a single diagnostic value.

5.6 Ethical implications in the education and training of health professionals

Since elastography is a relatively new technology, one of the bioethical challenges is to ensure that health professionals receive adequate and continuous training in its use. Lack of knowledge or adequate training in the use of elastography could lead to errors in diagnosis, which would compromise the quality of medical care and put patients' health at risk. It is essential that medical and educational institutions include specialized training in elastography, both in its technical handling and in the associated ethical considerations [18].

Professional organizations and health authorities should implement certification and recertification programs to ensure that health professionals who use elastography maintain high levels of competence. In addition, it is crucial that these programs include not only the technical aspect of the use of technology, but also the bioethical aspects, so that professionals can make ethical decisions in their daily clinical practice [20].

5.7 Use of artificial intelligence and machine learning techniques in elastography and ethical implications

The use of artificial intelligence (AI) and machine learning (ML) in elastography is revolutionizing the field of medical imaging, optimizing accuracy in the detection of tissue abnormalities and automating much of the analysis process. These technologies enable elastography systems to identify complex patterns that human eyes might miss, improving sensitivity and specificity in the detection of diseases such as liver fibrosis, cancer, and musculoskeletal diseases [30]. Furthermore, with the use of large volumes of data, ML algorithms can learn to distinguish subtle tissue features, which can increase diagnostic capability and reduce the time required to obtain results [31]. However, the integration of AI and ML in elastography raises serious ethical implications that must be addressed.

One of the main concerns is transparency in the algorithms used, as the automatic processes underlying clinical decision-making can be opaque to clinicians and, above all, to patients. This phenomenon, known as "algorithmic black box," implies that decisions influencing the diagnosis or treatment of patients could be made without users fully understanding the process [32]. This scenario raises questions about liability in case of diagnostic errors. Who is liable if the AI makes a failure, the physician or the system? Lack of clarity on these issues may affect the confidence of both healthcare professionals and patients.

Another key ethical consideration is equity in access to these advanced technologies. The implementation of AI and ML systems in elastography may be limited to high-resource medical centers, which could increase the gap in medical care between regions with different levels of infrastructure [33]. In addition, the use of data to train algorithms poses challenges in terms of privacy and information security, as large amounts of patient data are needed to feed ML systems, leading to the risk of exposure of sensitive data if not managed appropriately [34].

Therefore, it is essential that the development and implementation of AI and ML in elastography be accompanied by ethical regulations that ensure transparency, equity, and safety. Healthcare decision-makers should collaborate with ethicists and technology specialists to establish standards for the responsible use of these tools, always ensuring respect for patients' rights and quality of care.

6. Conclusion

Elastography, as an advanced medical imaging technique, has demonstrated a significant impact on the assessment of tissue elasticity, offering a valuable tool for the diagnosis and monitoring of various clinical conditions. Its technological evolution and its integration with new methodologies, such as AL and ML, promise to further improve its accuracy and applicability in clinical practice. These advances allow for higher resolution in the detection of tissue changes, as well as automation that can optimize the diagnostic process and reduce variability in the interpretation of results.

However, the development and implementation of elastography also face significant challenges, especially in the bioethical field. The protection of patient privacy, equity in access to technology, and transparency in the use of AL algorithms are critical aspects that must be addressed to ensure ethical and responsible practice. Standardization of procedures and continuous validation of techniques are essential to maintain quality and consistency in the application of elastography in different clinical settings.

Elastography education and training play a crucial role in overcoming these challenges. Adequate education and continuous updating in the use of this technology are essential to ensure that health professionals can use it effectively and ethically. The implementation of training curricula and the assessment of competence are necessary to maintain high standards in clinical practice and to improve the quality of patient care.

Looking to the future, elastography has the potential to further transform diagnostic medicine, but this requires a balanced approach that combines technological advancement with a strong ethical foundation. Collaboration between researchers, health professionals and regulatory bodies will be essential to address bioethical challenges and to promote responsible development and use of elastography. Only through this integrated approach can the benefits of this technology be maximized while minimizing risks and ensuring equitable, high-quality care for all patients.

Author details

Hector Fabio Restrepo-Guerrero
Department of Epidemiology and Bioethics, Institution Universidad Santo Tomas, Villavicencio, Colombia

*Address all correspondence to: restrepoguerrero@gmail.com

IntechOpen

References

[1] Oglat AA, Abunkhalil T. Ultrasound elastography: Methods, clinical applications, and limitations: A review article. Applied Sciences. 2024;**14**(10):4308

[2] Ricci P, Maggini E, Mancuso E, Lodise P, Cantisani V, Catalano C. Clinical application of breast elastography: State of the art. European Journal of Radiology. 2014;**83**(3):429-437

[3] Ozturk A, Grajo JR, Dhyani M, Anthony BW, Samir AE. Principles of ultrasound elastography. Abdominal Radiology. 2018;**43**(4):773-785

[4] Greenleaf JF. Ultrasound elastography: Development of novel technologies and standardization. Japanese Journal of Applied Physics. 2014;**53**(7):356-362

[5] Yoneda M, Honda Y, ogani A, Imajo K, Nakajima A. Advances in elastography techniques for liver disease. Journal of Medical Ultrasonics. 2020;**47**:521-533

[6] Sigrist RM, Liau J, Kaffas AE, Chammas MC, Willmann JK. Ultrasound elastography: Review of techniques and clinical applications. Theranostics. 2017;**7**(5):1303

[7] Beauchamp TL, Childress JF. Principles of Biomedical Ethics. Oxford University Press; 2001. ISBN 0195143310

[8] Gillon R. Medical ethics: Four principles plus attention to scope. BMJ. 1994;**309**(6948):184-188

[9] Campbell A. Bioethics: The Basics. Routledge; 2017. ISBN 978041579030

[10] Kass NE. An ethics framework for public health. American Journal of Public Health. 2001;**91**(11):1776-1782

[11] Daniels N. Just Health: Meeting Health Needs Fairly. Cambridge University Press; 2008. ISBN 970521699983

[12] Glover JJ. Ethical decision-making guidelines and tools. In: Ethical Challenges in the Management of Health Information. 2nd ed. Sudbury: Jones and Bartlett; 2006

[13] Jonsen A. Clinical Ethics: A Practical Approach to Ethical Decisions in Clinical Medicine. McGraw-Hill Education; 2015. ISBN 9780071845069

[14] Iserson KV. Principles of biomedical ethics. Emergency Medicine Clinics. 1999;**17**(2):283-306

[15] Beauchamp TL. Autonomy and consent. In: The Ethics of Consent: Theory and Practice. Oxford University Press; 2006. ISBN 9780195335149. Available from: https://doi.org/10.1093/acprof:oso/9780195335149.003.0003

[16] Faden RR, Beauchamp TL. A History and Theory of Informed Consent. Oxford University Press; 1986. ISBN: 9780195036862

[17] Greenhalgh T. How to Read a Paper: The Basics of Evidence-Based Medicine and Healthcare. 2nd ed. BMJ Books; 2019. ISBN 0-7279-1578-9

[18] Stokking R, Zubal IG, Viergever MA. Display of fused images: Methods, interpretation, and diagnostic improvements. Seminars in Nuclear Medicine. 2003;**33**(3):219-227

[19] Appelbaum PS, Berg JW, Lidz CW, Parker LS. Informed Consent: Legal Theory and Clinical Practice. Oxford University Press; 2001. ISBN 0195126777

[20] Niznick N, Lun R, Dewar B. Advanced consent for participation in acute care randomised control trials: Protocol for a scoping review. BMJ Open. 2020;**10**:244-252

[21] Daniels N, Sabin JE. Setting Limits Fairly: Can we Learn to Share Medical Resources? Oxford University Press; 2008. ISBN 9780195325959

[22] West RL. Social Justice: The Moral Foundations of Public Health and Health Policy. Oxford University Press; 2007. Available from: https://scholarship.law.georgetown.edu/facpub/789

[23] Greenhalgh T. How to Read a Paper: The Basics of Evidence-Based Medicine. BMJ Books; 2001. ISBN 0-7279-1578-9

[24] Benatar SR, Singer PA. A new look at international research ethics. BMJ. 2000;**321**(7264):824-826

[25] Emanuel EJ, Wendler D, Grady C. What makes clinical research ethical? Journal of the American Medical Association. 2000;**283**(20):2701-2711

[26] Resnik DB. The Ethics of Research with Human Subjects: Protecting People, Advancing Science, Promoting Integrity. Springer; 2018. ISBN: 9783319687551

[27] Morley J. The ethics of AI in medical imaging. The Journal of Ethics. 2020;**28**(3):245-256

[28] Ferraioli G. Performance of elastography in the diagnosis of liver fibrosis and liver Tumors. World Journal of Gastroenterology. 2012;**28**(3):245-256

[29] Coupier I. Role of elastography in rheumatic diseases. Current Opinion in Rheumatology. 2017;**29**(3):243-249

[30] Chartrand G, Cheng PM, Vorontsov E, Drozdzal M, Turcotte S, Pal CJ, et al. Deep learning: A primer for radiologists. Radiographics. 2017;**37**(7):2113-2131

[31] Lecun Y, Bengio Y, Hinton G. Deep learning. Nature. 2015;**521**(7553):436-444

[32] Pesapane F, Codari M, Sardanelli F. Artificial intelligence in medical imaging: Threat or opportunity? Radiologists again at the forefront of innovation in medicine. European Radiology Experimental. 2018;**1**(35). DOI: 10.1186/s41747-018-0061-6

[33] Topol EJ. High-performance medicine: The convergence of human and artificial intelligence. Nature Medicine. 2019;**25**(1):44-56

[34] Rieke N, Hancox J, Li W, Milletari F, Roth HR, Albarqouni S, et al. The future of digital health with federated learning. NPJ Digital Medicine. 2020;**3**(1):1-7

www.ingramcontent.com/pod-product-compliance
Lightning Source LLC
Chambersburg PA
CBHW081336190326
41458CB00018B/6024

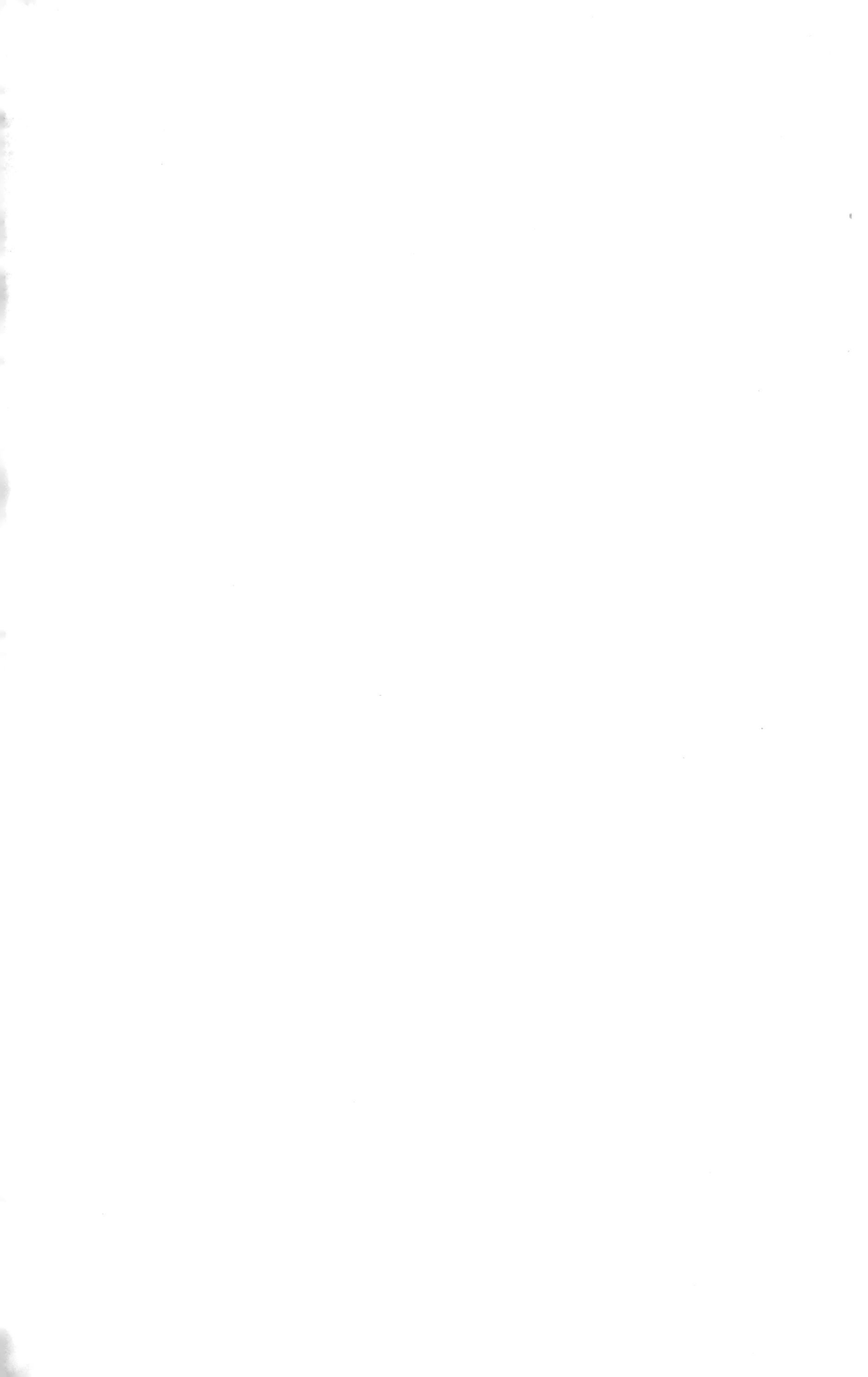